Respiratory Care Calculations

Third Edition

Exam #2 : 29, 85, 4, 34, 43, 52, 68

Exam #3 : 29, 31, 55, 74, 75, 76, 33, 55, 57, 63, 46, 84

Respiratory Care Calculations

Third Edition

David W. Chang, EdD, RRT-NPS

Professor
Department of Cardiorespiratory Care
University of South Alabama
Mobile, Alabama

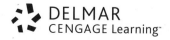

Australia • Brazil • Japan • Korea • Mexico • Singapore • Spain • United Kingdom • United States

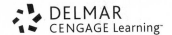

Title: Respiratory Care Calculations, Third Edition
Author David W. Chang

Vice President, Editorial: Dave Garza

Director of Learning Solutions: Matthew Kane

Senior Acquisitions Editor: Tari Broderick

Managing Editor: Marah Bellegarde

Associate Product Manager: Meghan E. Orvis

Editorial Assistant: Nicole Manikas

Vice President, Marketing: Jennifer Baker

Marketing Director: Wendy Mapstone

Marketing Manager: Jonathan Sheehan

Production Manager: Andrew Crouth

Senior Content Project Manager: Andrea Majot

Senior Art Director: Jack Pendleton

For product information and technology assistance, contact us at
Cengage Learning Customer & Sales Support, 1-800-354-9706
For permission to use material from this text or product,
submit all requests online at **www.cengage.com/permissions**
Further permissions questions can be emailed to
permissionrequest@cengage.com

Library of Congress Control Number: 2011934886

ISBN-13: 978-1-1113-0734-9

ISBN-10: 1-1113-0734-2

Delmar
5 Maxwell Drive
Clifton Park, NY 12065-2919
USA

Cengage Learning is a leading provider of customized learning solutions with office locations around the globe, including Singapore, the United Kingdom, Australia, Mexico, Brazil, and Japan. Locate your local office at:
international.cengage.com/region

Cengage Learning products are represented in Canada by Nelson Education, Ltd.

To learn more about Delmar, visit **www.cengage.com/delmar**

Purchase any of our products at your local college store or at our preferred online store **www.cengagebrain.com**

Printed in the United States of America
1 2 3 4 5 6 7 14 13 12 11

Dedicated to
my mother, Tsung-yuin,
my uncle Jim, and my wife, Bonnie

Contents

Section 3
Ventilator Waveform 245

Section 4
Basic Statistics and Educational Calculations 265

Section 5
Answer Key to Self-Assessment Questions 285

Section 6
Symbols and Abbreviations 293

Section 7
Units of Measurement 299

Listing of Appendices 309

Listing by Subject Areas

Introduction

The purpose of this book is to provide a clear and concise reference source for respiratory care calculations. It is intended for use in classroom, laboratory, and clinical settings by respiratory care students and practitioners.

Respiratory care equations are some of the most useful tools we use, directly or indirectly, in clinical practice. When an equation is correctly calculated, the data can be interpreted in a meaningful way. The patients we serve benefit from the proper application of clinical data.

WHY I WROTE THIS TEXT

In the first edition of this text, Dr. Donald F. Egan wrote in the Foreword about the pioneering days of *inhalation therapy*, "In that early phase of development, most therapists had a fearful opinion of mathematics, but fortunately arithmetic skills had little relevance to the work of most therapists—a far cry from today's needs." Dr. Egan's comment written in 1994 is certainly still accurate today. It is my sincere trust that respiratory therapists will continue to excel in the correct calculation and application of clinical data.

NEW TO THE THIRD EDITION

- Three new calculations: cerebral perfusion pressure, MDI/DPI dosage, and pressure support ventilation setting.
- All Self-Assessment Questions have been updated to reflect the examination format of the National Board for Respiratory Care (NBRC).
- The new section on ventilator waveforms provides detailed illustrations for most normal waveforms, as well as abnormal waveforms resulting from changing patient/ventilator conditions.
- More than double the number of appendices than the previous edition, with enhanced reference materials.
- Expanded number of calculation exercises and examples.

ORGANIZATION

The organization of this book represents the most user-friendly and easy-to-navigate layout on the market. Before the introduction of the respiratory care calculations is **Section 1**: Review of Basic Math Functions. This refresher of mathematical skills and concepts serves to ensure correct manipulation of numbers and variables in an equation.

Respiratory care calculations are presented alphabetically in **Section 2**, which allows the reader to locate specific calculations easily. For readers searching for calculations based on topic, a comprehensive Listing by Subject Area in the Table of Contents the includes appendices. In total, there are 85 useful calculations in this book.

Section 3: Ventilator Waveform has 26 different illustrations covering waveforms from volume-time to flow-volume waveforms. **Section 4**: Basic Statistics and Educational Calculations should be useful for educators and students. **Section 5** lists the answers to self-assessment questions. **Section 6** provides the Symbols and Abbreviations commonly used in respiratory care. **Section 7**: Units of Measurement allows the reader to make common conversions between different units of measurement. Concluding this book are 34 appendices in **Section 8** that cover clinical topics ranging from *Anatomical Values in Children and Adults* to *Weaning Criteria*.

FEATURES

Each calculation is presented with the **equation** followed by **normal values, examples,** and **exercises. References** are provided for each calculation section for further study. Supplemental information and clinical **notes** appear in the margin to provide additional explanation or clarification of the equation. Self-Assessment Questions, in NBRC format, can be found at the end of each calculation to enhance and reinforce learning and retention. **Answers** for these questions are listed in Section 5 of the book. With its comprehensive coverage of respiratory care calculations and extensive learning resources, readers will find this book useful in preparing for their laboratory and clinical practice.

About the Author

David W. Chang, EdD, RRT-NPS, is professor of cardiorespiratory care at the University of South Alabama in Mobile, Alabama. Over the years, he has served in different capacities in the American Association for Respiratory Care, Commission on Accreditation for Respiratory Care, and National Board for Respiratory Care. Dr. Chang has also authored *Clinical Application of Mechanical Ventilation* and created the rtexam.com Web site. He can be reached at dchang@usouthal.edu.

Acknowledgments

I would like to recognize my colleagues for their efforts in reviewing the manuscript during different stages of its development. They provided factual corrections and thoughtful comments and suggestions. The third edition would not be in its current form without their assistance. My deepest appreciation goes to:

Cynthia Annable, RRT-NPS, RPFT
Respiratory Therapy Program Director
Lake Superior College, Duluth, Minnesota

Dana Boomershine, BS, RRT
Program Coordinator of Respiratory Care
Trinity College of Nursing and Health Sciences
Rock Island, Illinosis

Lisa Conry, MA, RRT
Director of Clinical Education
Spartanburg Community College
Spartanburg, South Carolina

Rebecca Jeffs, DOM, RRT, RCP
Respiratory Therapy Program Director
Santa Fe Community College, Santa Fe, New Mexico

Lori Johnston, MEd, RRT
Director of Respiratory Care
Carrington College, Las Vegas, Nevada

J.K. LeJeune, MS, RRT, CPFT
Director of Respiratory Education
University of Arkansas Community College
Hope, Arkansas

Beth A. Zickefoose, BS, RRT-NPS, RPFT
Director of Clinical Education
Sinclair Community College, Dayton, Ohio

Publishing a textbook clearly involves many tedious steps, from conception of the contents to copyediting and printing the book. The team members at Delmar, Cengage Learning and S4 Carlisle Publishing Services made my job less challenging throughout the process. I could not begin to describe how each of them attended to all the necessary details for the production of the third edition of *Respiratory Care Calculations*. For each individual's diligent effort. I thank:

Tari Broderick
Senior Acquisitions Editor

Meghan E. Orvis
Associate Product Manager

Andrea Majot
Senior Content Project Manager

Nicole Manikas
Editorial Assistant

Allison Frank Esposito
Copy Editor

1

Review of
Basic Math Functions

Review of
Basic Math Functions

1. Add numbers with decimals.
   Note: Line up the decimals properly.

EXAMPLE $43.45 + 10.311 + 0.25 = 54.011$

$$\begin{array}{r} 43.45 \\ 10.311 \\ +\ 0.25 \\ \hline 54.011 \end{array}$$

2. Subtract numbers with decimals.
   Note: Line up the decimals properly.

EXAMPLE $198.24 - 40.015 = 158.225$

$$\begin{array}{r} 198.24 \\ -\ 40.015 \\ \hline 158.225 \end{array}$$

3. Multiply numbers with decimals.
   Note: Count the total number of digits after the decimals in the numbers and place the decimal in the answer accordingly.

EXAMPLE $50.6 \times 0.002 = 0.1012$ can be treated as

$$\begin{array}{r} 506 \\ \times\ \ 2 \\ \hline 1{,}012 \end{array}$$

There are a total of 4 digits (1 in 50.6 + 3 in 0.002) after the decimals in the numbers. The decimal in the product 1,012 comes after the 2 (1,012 = 1,012.0); moving it 4 places to the left gives an answer of 0.1012.

4. Divide numbers with decimals.

Terminology: $\dfrac{\text{Dividend}}{\text{Divisor}} = \text{Answer}$

Step 1. Count and compare the number of digits after the decimal in the dividend and after the decimal in the divisor.

Step 2. Move the decimal points for both dividend and divisor to the right so that they become whole numbers. Remember to move decimals the same number of places to the right in both the dividend and divisor.

EXAMPLE $\dfrac{0.68}{3.4}$ can be changed to $\dfrac{68}{340} = 0.2$

Move the decimal points two places to the right for both the dividend and the divisor (0.68 is changed to 68 and 3.4 is changed to 340).

EXAMPLE $\dfrac{2.4}{0.006}$ can be changed to $\dfrac{2,400}{6} = 400$

Move the decimal points three places to the right for the dividend and the divisor (2.4 is changed to 2,400 and 0.006 is changed to 6).

5. Add/subtract and multiply/divide
    Note: Perform multiplication/division **before** addition/subtraction.

EXAMPLE 1
$$12 \times 6 - 2 = (12 \times 6) - 2$$
$$= 72 - 2$$
$$= 70$$

EXAMPLE 2
$$116 - \dfrac{455}{5} = 116 - \left(\dfrac{455}{5}\right)$$
$$= 116 - 91$$
$$= 25$$

6. Parentheses
    Note: Perform calculation within parentheses in the order ( ), [ ], and { }.

EXAMPLE 1
$$12 \times (6 - 2) = 12 \times 4$$
$$= 48$$

EXAMPLE 2
$$194 - \{[20 \times (9 - 5)] + 14\} = 194 - \{[20 \times 4] + 14\}$$
$$= 194 - \{80 + 14\}$$
$$= 194 - 94$$
$$= 100$$

7. Ratio
    Note: A ratio compares two related quantities or measurements. It is usually expressed in the form 1:2, as in *I*:*E* ratio.

EXAMPLE 1   *I*:*E* ratio of 1:2 means that the expiratory phase (*E*) is two times as long as the inspiratory phase (*I*). A ratio is dimensionless: it does not include units such as seconds or inches. An *I*:*E* ratio of 1:2 may mean that the inspiratory time (*I* time) is 1 second and expiratory time (*E* time) is 2 seconds *or* the *I* time is 2 seconds and the *E* time is 4 seconds.

EXAMPLE 2   Inverse *I*:*E* ratio of 2:1 means that the inspiratory phase is two times as long as the expiratory phase.

EXAMPLE 3   Oxygen: air entrainment ratio of 1:4 means that 1 part of oxygen is combined with 4 parts of air.

8.   Percentage

Note: Percentage expresses a value in parts of 100. It is written in the form 65% or 0.65, as in F_IO_2.

EXAMPLE 1   An intrapulmonary shunt of 15% means that 15 of 100 units of perfusion do not take part in gas exchange.

EXAMPLE 2   An arterial oxygen content of 21 vol% means that 21 of 100 units of arterial blood are saturated with oxygen.

9.   Relationships of X and Y in equation $A = \dfrac{X^*}{Y}$

[When A is constant, X and Y are directly related]

EXAMPLE 1 $\text{Resistance} = \dfrac{\text{Pressure change } (\Delta P)}{\text{Flow}}$

When airway resistance is constant, an **increase** in driving pressure generates a **higher** flow. Likewise, a **decrease** in driving pressure yields a **lower** flow.

EXAMPLE 2 $\text{Compliance} = \dfrac{\text{Volume change } (\Delta V)}{\text{Pressure change } (\Delta P)}$

When compliance is constant, an **increase** in pressure generates a **higher** lung volume. By the same token, a **decrease** in pressure **lowers** the lung volume.

10.   Relationships of A and X in equation $A = \dfrac{X}{Y}$

[When Y is constant, A and X are directly related]

EXAMPLE 1 $\text{Resistance} = \dfrac{\text{Pressure change } (\Delta P)}{\text{Flow}}$

In order to maintain a constant flow, an **increase** in driving pressure is needed to overcome a **higher** resistance. If the resistance is **low, less** pressure is needed to maintain a constant flow.

EXAMPLE 2 $\text{Compliance} = \dfrac{\text{Volume change } (\Delta V)}{\text{Pressure change } (\Delta P)}$

When a constant peak inspiratory pressure is used on a pressure-limited ventilator (e.g., IPPB), the volume delivered is **increased** in the presence of **high** compliance. On the other hand, the volume delivered by a pressure-limited ventilator is **decreased** with **low** compliance.

11.   Relationships of A and Y in equation $A = \dfrac{X}{Y}$

[When X is constant, A and Y are inversely related]

$A = \dfrac{X}{Y}$ can be rewritten as $X = AY$ or $Y = \dfrac{X}{A}$. When any two of three values are known, the third can be calculated.

EXAMPLE 1

$$\text{Resistance} = \frac{\text{Pressure change } (\Delta P)}{\text{Flow}}$$

In the presence of **increasing** airway resistance, air flow to the lungs is **decreased** if the pressure (work of breathing or ventilator work) remains constant. On the other hand, with **decreasing** airway resistance, air flow to the lungs is **increased** at constant pressure (work of breathing or ventilator work).

EXAMPLE 2

$$\text{Compliance} = \frac{\text{Volume change } (\Delta V)}{\text{Pressure change } (\Delta P)}$$

During volume-controlled ventilation, the peak inspiratory pressure of the ventilator **increases** in the presence of **decreasing** compliance. As the compliance **improves** (**increases**), the inspiratory pressure **decreases**.

12.   Relationships of A, B and X, Y in equation $\dfrac{A}{B} = \dfrac{X}{Y}$ [same as $AY = BX$]

[A or Y is directly related to B or X. A and Y are inversely related to each other]
[B or X is directly related to A or Y. B and X are inversely related to each other]

2

Respiratory Care Calculations

1

Airway Resistance: Estimated (R_{aw})

This equation estimates the airway resistance of an intubated patient on a volume ventilator. (PIP-P_{PLAT}) represents the pressure gradient in the presence of flow.

In ventilators with constant flow patterns, the inspiratory flow rate can be used in this equation. Otherwise, a pneumotachometer may be needed to measure the inspiratory flow rate at PIP. Flow rates in L/min should first be changed to L/sec by dividing L/min by 60. For example:

$$40 \text{ L/min} = \frac{40(L/min)}{60}$$
$$= 0.67 \text{ L/sec}$$

Some conditions leading to an increase in airway resistance include bronchospasm, retained secretions, and use of a small endotracheal or tracheostomy tube. These increases in airway resistance can be minimized by using bronchodilators for bronchospasm, frequent suctioning for retained secretions, and the largest appropriate endotracheal or tracheostomy tube.

EQUATION

$$R_{aw} = \frac{\left(PIP - P_{PLAT}\right)^*}{Flow}$$

R_{aw} : Airway resistance in cm H_2O/L/sec

PIP : Peak inspiratory pressure in cm H_2O

P_{PLAT} : Plateau pressure in cm H_2O (static pressure)

Flow : Flow rate in L/sec

NORMAL VALUE

0.6 to 2.4 cm H_2O/L/sec at flow rate of 0.5 L/sec (30 L/min). If the patient is intubated, use serial measurements to establish trend.

EXAMPLE

Calculate the estimated airway resistance of a patient whose peak inspiratory pressure is 25 cm H_2O and whose plateau pressure is 10 cm H_2O. The ventilator flow rate is set at 60 L/min (1 L/sec).

$$R_{aw} = \frac{\left(PIP - P_{PLAT}\right)}{Flow}$$
$$= \frac{\left(25 - 10\right)}{1}$$
$$= \frac{15}{1}$$
$$= 15 \text{ cm } H_2O\text{/L/sec}$$

EXERCISE

Given: Peak inspiratory pressure = 45 cm H_2O
Plateau pressure = 35 cm H_2O
Inspiratory flow = 50 L/min (0.83 L/sec)

Calculate the estimated airway resistance.

[Answer: R_{aw} = 12 cm H_2O/L/sec]

REFERENCE

Wilkins (2)

*In nonintubated subjects, a body plethysmography must be used to measure and calculate the airway resistance by

$$R_{aw} = \frac{\left(P_{ao} - P_{alv}\right)}{Flow},$$ where P_{ao} is the pressure at the airway

opening and P_{alv} is the alveolar pressure.

SELF-ASSESSMENT QUESTIONS

1a. When volume-controlled ventilation is used, the $(PIP - P_{PLAT})$ gradient is directly related to the:

  (A) patient's airway resistance.
  (B) frequency.
  (C) F_IO_2.
  (D) patient's lung compliance.

1b. Calculate the estimated airway resistance ($R_{aw_{est}}$) of a patient whose peak inspiratory pressure is 60 cm H_2O and plateau pressure is 40 cm H_2O. The ventilator constant flow rate is set at 60 L/min (1 L/sec).

  (A) 10 cm H_2O/L/sec
  (B) 20 cm H_2O/L/sec
  (C) 50 cm H_2O/L/sec
  (D) 100 cm H_2O/L/sec

$$\frac{60 - 40}{1} = \frac{20}{1} = 20 \text{ cm } H_2O/L/sec$$

1c. Given: PIP = 60 cm H_2O, P_{PLAT} = 40 cm H_2O, $PEEP$ = 10 cm H_2O. Calculate the estimated R_{aw} if the constant flow rate is 50 L/min (0.83 L/sec).

  (A) 20 cm H_2O/L/sec
  (B) 24 cm H_2O/L/sec
  (C) 28 cm H_2O/L/sec
  (D) 32 cm H_2O/L/sec

$$\frac{60 - 40}{0.83 L/sec} = \frac{20}{0.8 L/sec} = 24.09$$

Chapter

2

Alveolar–Arterial Oxygen Tension Gradient: $P(A - a)O_2$

NOTE

The value of $P(A - a)O_2$ (also known as $A - a$ gradient) can be used to estimate (1) the degree of hypoxemia and (2) the degree of physiologic shunt. It is derived from a less commonly used shunt equation:

$$\frac{Q_s}{Q_T} = \frac{(P_A O_2 - P_a O_2 \times 0.003)}{(C_a O_2 - C_{\bar{v}} O_2) + (P_A O_2 - P_a O_2) \times 0.003}$$

The $P(A - a)O_2$ is increased when hypoxemia results from $\frac{V}{Q}$ mismatch, diffusion defect, or shunt. In the absence of cardiopulmonary disease, it increases with aging.

EQUATION

$$P(A - a)O_2 = P_A O_2 - P_a O_2$$

$P(A - a)O_2$: Alveolar-arterial oxygen tension gradient in mm Hg

$P_A O_2$: Alveolar-arterial oxygen tension in mm Hg*

$P_a O_2$: Arterial oxygen tension in mm Hg

NORMAL VALUE

(1) On *room* air, the $P(A - a)O_2$ should be less than 4 mm Hg for every 10 years in age. For example, the $P(A - a)O_2$ should be less than 24 mm Hg for a 60-year-old patient.

(2) On *100% oxygen*, every 50 mm Hg difference in $P(A - a)O_2$ approximates 2% shunt.

EXAMPLE 1

Given: $P_A O_2$ = 100 mm Hg

$P_a O_2$ = 85 mm Hg

$F_I O_2$ = 21%

Patient age = 40 years

Calculate $P(A - a)O_2$. Is it abnormal for this patient?

$P(A - a)O_2$ = $P_A O_2 - P_a O_2$

= (100 − 85) mm Hg

= 15 mm Hg

$P(A - a)O_2$ of 15 mm Hg is normal for a 40-year-old patient.

EXAMPLE 2

Given: $P_A O_2$ = 660 mm Hg

$P_a O_2$ = 360 mm Hg

$F_I O_2$ = 100%

Calculate $P(A - a)O_2$. What is the estimated physiologic shunt in percent?

$P(A - a)O_2$ = $P_A O_2 - P_a O_2$

= (660 − 360) mm Hg

= 300 mm Hg

* See Alveolar Oxygen Tension ($P_A O_2$) for calculation of $P_A O_2$.

Since every 50 mm Hg difference in $P(A - a)O_2$ approximates 2% shunt, 300 mm Hg $P(A - a)O_2$ difference is estimated to be 12% shunt:

$$50 \text{ mm Hg} = 2\%$$

$$\frac{50 \text{ mm Hg}}{300 \text{ mm Hg}} = \frac{2\%}{x\%}$$

$$x = \frac{2 \times 300}{50}\%$$

$$= \frac{600}{50}\%$$

$$= 12\%$$

EXERCISE 1

Given: P_AO_2 = 93 mm Hg
 P_aO_2 = 60 mm Hg
 F_IO_2 = 21%
 Patient age = 65 years

Calculate $P(A - a)O_2$.

Is the $P(A - a)O_2$ normal or abnormal based on the patient's age?

[Answer: $P(A - a)O_2$ = 33 mm Hg. It is abnormal because 33 mm Hg is more than 26 mm Hg, the allowable difference for patient's age.]

EXERCISE 2

Given: P_AO_2 = 646 mm Hg
 P_aO_2 = 397 mm Hg
 F_IO_2 = 100%

Calculate the $P(A - a)O_2$ and estimate the percent physiologic shunt.

[Answer: $P(A - a)O_2$ = 249 mm Hg. The estimated shunt is 10% because every 50 mm Hg $P(A - a)O_2$ difference represents about 2% shunt:

$$50 \text{ mm Hg} = 2\%$$

$$\frac{50 \text{ mm Hg}}{249 \text{ mm Hg}} = \frac{2\%}{x\%}$$

$$x = \frac{2 \times 249}{50}\%$$

$$= \frac{498}{50}\%$$

$$= 9.96\% \text{ or } 10\%$$

REFERENCES

Shapiro; Wilkins (2)

SEE

Arterial-Alveolar Oxygen Tension (a/A) Ratio.

SELF-ASSESSMENT QUESTIONS

2a. Given the following values for room air: $P_AO_2 = 105$ mm Hg, $P_aO_2 = 70$ mm Hg. What is the $P(A - a)O_2$? Is it normal for a 70-year-old patient?

(A) 70 mm Hg; normal

(B) 70 mm Hg; abnormal

(C) 35 mm Hg; normal

(D) 35 mm Hg; abnormal

2b. If a patient's P_aO_2 is 70 mm Hg and $P(A - a)O_2$ is 30 mm Hg, what is the P_AO_2?

(A) 30 mm Hg

(B) 40 mm Hg

(C) 70 mm Hg

(D) 100 mm Hg

2c. Given: $P_AO_2 = 638$ mm Hg, $P_aO_2 = 240$ mm Hg, $F_IO_2 = 100\%$. What is the calculated $P(A - a)O_2$ and the estimated physiologic shunt?

(A) 240 mm Hg; 12%

(B) 240 mm Hg; 16%

(C) 398 mm Hg; 16%

(D) 398 mm Hg; 22%

2d. A patient has a P_aO_2 of 540 mm Hg on 100% oxygen. If the P_AO_2 is 642 mm Hg, what is the alveolar-arterial oxygen tension difference? What is the estimated shunt based on this difference?

(A) 102 mm Hg; 2%

(B) 102 mm Hg; 4%

(C) 540 mm Hg; 4%

(D) 540 mm Hg; 8%

Chapter

3

Alveolar Oxygen Tension (P_AO_2)

NOTE

P_AO_2 is primarily used for other calculations such as alveolar-arterial oxygen tension gradient ($A - a$ gradient) and arterial/alveolar oxygen tension (a/A) ratio. The P_AO_2 value is directly proportional to the F_IO_2. Under normal conditions, a higher F_IO_2 gives a higher P_AO_2 value and vice versa.

EQUATION

$$P_AO_2 = (P_B - P_{H_2O}) \times F_IO_2 - (P_aCO_2 \times 1.25)*$$

P_AO_2 : Alveolar oxygen tension in mm Hg
P_B : Barometric pressure in mm Hg
P_{H_2O} : Water vapor pressure, 47 mm Hg saturated at 37 °C
F_IO_2 : Inspired oxygen concentration in percent
P_aCO_2 : Arterial carbon dioxide tension in mm Hg
1.25 : $\dfrac{1}{0.8}\left(\dfrac{1}{\text{Normal respiratory exchange ratio}}\right)$;

* This ratio is omitted when F_IO_2 is greater than 60%.

NORMAL VALUE

The normal values vary according to the F_IO_2.

EXAMPLE

Given: P_B = 760 mm Hg
P_{H_2O} = 47 mm Hg
F_IO_2 = 40% or 0.4
P_aCO_2 = 30 mm Hg
P_AO_2 = $(P_B - P_{H_2O}) \times F_IO_2 - (P_aCO_2 \times 1.25)$
= $(760 - 47) \times 0.4 - (30 \times 1.25)$
= $713 \times 0.4 - 37.5$
= $285.2 - 37.5$
= 247.7 or 248 mm Hg

EXERCISE

Given: P_B = 750 mm Hg
P_{H_2O} = 47 mm Hg
F_IO_2 = 50% or 0.5
P_aCO_2 = 40 mm Hg

Calculate the P_AO_2.

[Answer: P_AO_2 = 301.5 or 302 mm Hg]

*Modified from: $P_AO_2 = (P_B - P_{H_2O}) \times F_IO_2 - P_aCO_2 \times$

$[F_IO_2 + \dfrac{(1 - F_IO_2)}{R}]$, where R is the respiratory exchange ratio, normally 0.8.

REFERENCES	Shapiro (1); Wilkins (2)
SEE	*Appendix X, $P_{A}O_2$ at Selected $F_{I}O_2$; and Appendix Y, Partial Pressure (in mm Hg) of Gases in the Air, Alveoli, and Blood*

SELF-ASSESSMENT QUESTIONS

3a. Which of the following is the clinical equation to calculate the partial pressure of oxygen in the alveoli?

    (A) $P_{A}O_2 = (P_{B} - P_{H_2O}) \times F_{I}O_2 - (P_{a}CO_2 \times 1.25)$
    (B) $P_{A}O_2 = (P_{B} - P_{H_2O}) \times F_{I}O_2$
    (C) $P_{A}O_2 = (P_{B} \times F_{I}O_2) - (P_{a}CO_2 - P_{H_2O})$
    (D) $P_{A}O_2 = (P_{B} \times F_{I}O_2) - P_{H_2O}$

3b. Given: $P_{B} = 760$ mm Hg, $P_{H_2O} = 47$ mm Hg, $F_{I}O_2 = 0.7$, $P_{a}CO_2 = 50$ mm Hg. The $P_{A}O_2$ is about (Do not use respiratory exchange ratio in equation because $F_{I}O_2$ is greater than 60%.)

    (A) 403 mm Hg
    (B) 417 mm Hg
    (C) 428 mm Hg
    (D) 449 mm Hg

3c. Calculate the alveolar oxygen tension ($P_{A}O_2$), given the following values: $P_{B} = 750$ mm Hg, $P_{H_2O} = 47$ mm Hg, $F_{I}O_2 = 30\%$ or 0.3, and $P_{a}CO_2 = 40$ mm Hg.

    (A) 30 mm Hg
    (B) 100 mm Hg
    (C) 161 mm Hg
    (D) 170 mm Hg

3d. Given: $P_{B} = 760$ mm Hg, $P_{H_2O} = 47$ mm Hg, $F_{I}O_2 = 70\%$ or 0.7, and $P_{a}CO_2 = 40$ mm Hg. What is the calculated alveolar oxygen tension ($P_{A}O_2$)? (Do not use respiratory exchange ratio in equation since $F_{I}O_2$ is greater than 60%.)

    (A) 70 mm Hg
    (B) 100 mm Hg
    (C) 449 mm Hg
    (D) 459 mm Hg

Chapter

4

Anion Gap

NOTES

Anion gap helps to evaluate the overall electrolyte balance between the cations and anions in the extracellular fluid. Potassium is not included in the calculation because it contributes little to the extracellular cation concentration. If potassium is included in the equation, the normal value range would be 15 to 20 mEq/L.

Metabolic acidosis in the presence of a *normal anion gap* is usually caused by a loss of base. It is known as hyperchloremia metabolic acidosis because this condition is usually related to loss of HCO_3^- and accumulation of chloride ions.

Metabolic acidosis in the presence of an *increased anion gap* is usually the result of increased fixed acids. These fixed acids may be produced (e.g., renal failure, diabetic ketoacidosis, lactic acidosis), or they may be added to the body (e.g., poisoning by salicylates, methanol, and ethylene glycol).

Fluid and electrolyte therapy is indicated when there is a significant anion gap (> 16 mEq/L).

EQUATION

$$\text{Anion gap} = Na^+ - (Cl^- + HCO_3^-)$$

Na^+ : Serum sodium concentration in mEq/L
Cl^- : Serum chloride concentration in mEq/L
HCO_3^- : Serum bicarbonate concentration in mEq/L

NORMAL VALUE

10 to 14 mEq/L
15 to 20 mEq/L if potassium (K^+) is included in the equation

EXAMPLE

Given: Na^+ = 140 mEq/L
Cl^- = 105 mEq/L
HCO_3^- = 22 mEq/L
Calculate the anion gap.

$$
\begin{aligned}
\text{Anion gap} &= Na^+ - (Cl^- + HCO_3^-) \\
&= 140 - (105 + 22) \\
&= 140 - 127 \\
&= 13 \text{ mEq/L}
\end{aligned}
$$

EXERCISE

Given: Na^+ = 130 mEq/L
Cl^- = 92 mEq/L
HCO_3^- = 20 mEq/L
What is the calculated anion gap?

[Answer: Anion gap = 18 mEq/L]

REFERENCE

Wilkins (1)

SEE

Appendix J, Electrolyte Concentrations in Plasma

SELF-ASSESSMENT QUESTIONS

4a. A physician asks the therapist to evaluate a patient's overall status of electrolyte balance. The therapist should use the following set of electrolyes to calculate the anion gap:

(A) Na^+, H^+, Cl^-, HCO_3^-
(B) Na^+, K^+, HCO_3^-
(C) Na^+, Cl^-, HCO_3^-
(D) Na^+, Ca^{++}, Cl^-, HCO_3^-

4b. Given: $Na^+ = 138$ mEq/L, $Cl^- = 102$ mEq/L, $HCO_3^- = 25$ mEq/L. Calculate the anion gap.

(A) 36 mEq/L
(B) 25 mEq/L
(C) 12 mEq/L
(D) 11 mEq/L

4c. Given: $Na^+ = 135$ mEq/L, $Cl^- = 96$ mEq/L, $HCO_3^- = 22$ mEq/L. What is the calculated anion gap?

(A) 15 mEq/L
(B) 17 mEq/L
(C) 20 mEq/L
(D) 22 mEq/L

4d. Metabolic acidosis with a normal anion gap is typically caused by a:

(A) gain of acid.
(B) gain of base.
(C) loss of acid.
(D) loss of base.

4e. Metabolic acidosis with an increased anion gap is usually the result of:

(A) increased fixed acid.
(B) increased fixed base.
(C) decreased fixed acid.
(D) decreased fixed base.

Chapter

5

Arterial/Alveolar Oxygen Tension (a/A) Ratio

NOTE

The a/A ratio is an indicator of the efficiency of oxygen transport. A low a/A ratio reflects ventilation/perfusion (V/Q) mismatch, diffusion defect, or shunt.

This ratio is often used to calculate the approximate F_IO_2 needed to obtain a desired P_aO_2.

EQUATION

$$a/A \text{ ratio} = \frac{P_aO_2}{P_AO_2}$$

a/A ratio	:	Arterial/alveolar oxygen tension ratio in percent
P_aO_2	:	Arterial oxygen tension in mm Hg
P_AO_2	:	Alveolar oxygen tension in mm Hg*

NORMAL VALUE

$> 60\%$

EXAMPLE

Calculate the a/A ratio if the $P_aO_2 = 100$ mm Hg and $P_AO_2 = 248$ mm Hg.

$$a/A \text{ ratio} = \frac{P_aO_2}{P_AO_2}$$

$$= \frac{100}{248}$$

$$= 0.403 \text{ or } 40\%$$

EXERCISE

Given: $P_AO_2 = 320$ mm Hg
$P_aO_2 = 112$ mm Hg
Calculate the a/A ratio.

[Answer: a/A ratio $= 0.35$ or 35%]

REFERENCE

Wilkins (2)

SEE

Alveolar – Arterial Oxygen Tension Gradient: $P(A - a)O_2$;
F_IO_2 Needed for a Desired P_aO_2.

Refer to Alveolar Oxygen Tension (P_AO_2) for calculation of P_AO_2.

SELF-ASSESSMENT QUESTIONS

5a. Calculate the a/A ratio if the P_aO_2 = 80 mm Hg and P_AO_2 = 170 mm Hg.

    (A) 47%

    (B) 80%

    (C) 21%

    (D) 210%

5b. Given: P_AO_2 = 210 mm Hg, P_aO_2 = 45 mm Hg. Calculate the a/A ratio.

    (A) 12%

    (B) 21%

    (C) 30%

    (D) 47%

5c. Ventilation and perfusion defects may lead to a(n):

    (A) increased P_aO_2.

    (B) increased P_AO_2.

    (C) decreased a/A ratio.

    (D) increased a/A ratio.

5d. In the a/A ratio calculation, the P_AO_2 is:

    (A) determined by the ventilation.

    (B) determined by the perfusion.

    (C) a calculated value.

    (D) usually lower than the P_aO_2.

6

Arterial–Mixed Venous Oxygen Content Difference $[C(a-\bar{v})O_2]$

NOTES

Measurements of arterial mixed venous oxygen content difference $[C(a-\bar{v})O_2]$ are useful in assessing changes in oxygen consumption and cardiac output. Under conditions of normal oxygen consumption and cardiac output, about 25% of the available oxygen is used for tissue metabolism. Therefore, a $C(a-\bar{v})O_2$ of 5 vol% (C_aO_2 20 vol%$-C_{\bar{v}}O_2$ 15 vol%) reflects a balanced relationship between oxygen consumption and cardiac output (Figure 2-1).

According to the cardiac output equation (Fick's estimated method)

$$\dot{Q}_T = \frac{\dot{V}O_2}{\left[C(a-\bar{v})O_2\right]}$$

the arterial-mixed venous oxygen content difference $[C(a-\bar{v})O_2]$ is directly related to the oxygen consumption ($\dot{V}O_2$) and inversely related to the cardiac output ($\dot{Q}_T$).

Relationship of $C(a-\bar{v})O_2$ and oxygen consumption

If the *cardiac output* stays unchanged or is unable to compensate for hypoxia, an increase of oxygen consumption (metabolic rate) will cause an increase in $C(a-\bar{v})O_2$. A decrease of oxygen consumption will cause a decrease in $C(a-\bar{v})O_2$.

EQUATION

$$C\left(a-\bar{v}\right)O_2 = C_aO_2 - C_{\bar{v}}O_2$$

$C\left(a-\bar{v}\right)O_2$: Arterial − mixed venous oxygen content difference in vol%

C_aO_2 : Arterial oxygen content in vol%

$C_{\bar{v}}O_2$: Mixed venous oxygen content in vol%

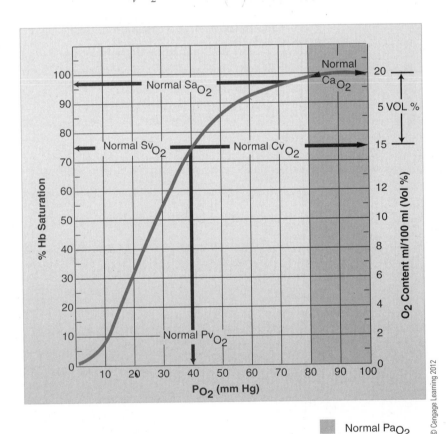

© Cengage Learning 2012

Figure 2-1 Oxygen dissociation curve. The normal oxygen content difference between arterial and venous blood is about 5 vol%. Note that both the right side and the left side of the graph illustrate that approximately 25% of the available oxygen is used for tissue metabolism, and the hemoglobin returning to the lungs is normally about 75% saturated with oxygen.

NOTES *(continued)*

Relationship of $C(a-\bar{v})O_2$ and cardiac output

When *oxygen consumption* remains constant, the $C(a-\bar{v})O_2$ becomes a good indicator of the cardiac output. A decrease

of $C(a-\bar{v})O_2$ is indicative of an increase of cardiac output, and an increase of $C(a-\bar{v})O_2$ reflects a decrease of cardiac output.

For a summary of factors that change the $C(a-\bar{v})O_2$ values, see Tables 2-1 and 2-2.

TABLE 2-1 Factors That Increase the $C(a-\bar{v})O_2$

Decreased cardiac output

Periods of increased oxygen consumption

  Exercise

  Seizures

  Shivering

  Hyperthermia

TABLE 2-2 Factors That Decrease the $C(a-\bar{v})O_2$

Increased cardiac output

Skeletal muscle relaxation (e.g., induced by drugs)

Peripheral shunting (e.g., sepsis, trauma)

Certain poisons (e.g., cyanide prevents cellular metabolism)

Hypothermia

NORMAL VALUES

<5 vol% for healthy or critically ill patients with cardiovascular compensation.

>6 vol% for critically ill patients without cardiovascular compensation.

EXAMPLE

Given:
$$C_aO_2 = 18.3 \text{ vol}\%$$
$$C_{\bar{v}}O_2 = 14.1 \text{ vol}\%$$
$$C(a-\bar{v})O_2 = C_aO - C_{\bar{v}}O_2$$
$$= 18.3 - 14.1$$
$$= 4.2 \text{ vol}\%$$

EXERCISE 1

Given: $C_aO_2 = 16.2 \text{ vol}\%$

$C_{\bar{v}}O_2 = 13.1 \text{ vol}\%$

Calculate the $C(a-\bar{v})O_2$. Is it normal for a critically ill patient?

[Answer: $C(a-\bar{v})O_2 = 3.1$ vol%. Normal for this patient.]

EXERCISE 2

Given: $C_aO_2 = 16.8 \text{ vol}\%$
$C_{\bar{v}}O_2 = 10.6 \text{ vol}\%$
Calculate the $C(a-\bar{v})O_2$. Is it normal for a critically ill patient?

[Answer: $C(a-\bar{v})O_2 = 6.2$ vol%. Abnormal for this patient.]

REFERENCE

Des Jardins

SEE

Oxygen Content: Arterial (C_aO_2); Oxygen Content: Mixed Venous $\left(C_{\bar{v}}O_2\right)$; Appendix V, Oxygen Transport.

SELF-ASSESSMENT QUESTIONS

6a. The normal arterial-mixed venous oxygen content difference $\left[C\left(a-\bar{v}\right)O_2\right]$ is or less.

(A) 20 vol%

(B) 15 vol%

(C) 10 vol%

(D) 5 vol%

6b. A critically ill patient has the following oxygen content measurements: $C_aO_2 = 20.5$ vol%, $C_{\bar{v}}O_2 = 16.6$ vol%. What is the arterial-mixed venous oxygen content difference $\left[C\left(a-\bar{v}\right)O_2\right]$? Is it normal for this patient?

(A) 3.9 vol%; normal

(B) 3.9 vol%; abnormal

(C) 37.1 vol%; normal

(D) 37.1 vol%; abnormal

6c. The following oxygen content measurements are obtained from a critically ill patient: $C_cO_2 = 21.0$ vol%, $C_aO_2 = 19.8$ vol%, $C_{\bar{v}}O_2 = 12.8$ vol%. What is the calculated arterial-mixed venous oxygen content difference $\left[C\left(a-\bar{v}\right)O_2\right]$? Is it normal for this patient?

(A) 0.2 vol%; normal

(B) 0.2 vol%; abnormal

(C) 7 vol%; normal

(D) 7 vol%; abnormal

Chapter

7

ATPS to BTPS

NOTE

According to Charles' law, lung volumes and flow rates measured at room temperature should be corrected to reflect the actual values at body temperature. The conversion factors in Appendix F should be used if the pulmonary function device does not correct for the temperature change.

The values shown in Appendix F are accurate for a barometric pressure of 760 mm Hg. At barometric pressures as low as 750 mm Hg, changes in the conversion factors are negligible. If a precise conversion factor is desired at any barometric pressure, use the equation included in Appendix F.

EQUATION

$$\text{Volume}_{BTPS} = \text{Volume}_{ATPS} \times \text{Factor}$$

Volume_{BTPS} : Gas volume saturated with water at body temperature (37°C) and ambient pressure

Volume_{ATPS} : Gas volume saturated with water at ambient (room) temperature and pressure

Factor : Factors for converting gas volumes from ATPS to BTPS (Appendix F)

EXAMPLE

A tidal volume measured under the ATPS condition is 600 mL. What is the corrected volume if the room temperature is 25°C?

$$\text{Volume}_{BTPS} = \text{Volume}_{ATPS} \times \text{Factor at ambient temperature}$$
$$= \text{Volume} \times \text{Factor at } 25°C$$
$$= 600 \times 1.075 \text{ (Appendix F)}$$
$$= 645 \text{ mL}$$

EXERCISE 1

A tidal volume was recorded at 23°C. What should be the factor for converting this measurement from ATPS to BTPS at normal body temperature (37°C)?

[Answer: Conversion factor = 1.085]

EXERCISE 2

A peak flow of 120 L/min was recorded at 27°C. What is the corrected flow rate at body temperature (37°C)?

[Answer: Flow rate = 127.56 or 128 L/min]

REFERENCE

Wilkins (2)

SELF-ASSESSMENT QUESTIONS

7a. What is the conversion factor from ATPS to BTPS at 26°C?

(A) 1.068
(B) 1.063
(C) 1.075
(D) 1.000

7b. The vital capacity (VC) measured under ATPS conditions is 3,600 mL. What is the corrected VC at BTPS if the measurement was done at 27°C? (Conversion factor from 27 to 37°C is 1.063.)

(A) 360 mL
(B) 3,000 mL
(C) 3,387 mL
(D) 3,827 mL

7c. An average tidal volume (V_T) of 580 mL was recorded under ATPS conditions. If the ambient temperature at the time of measurement is 25°C, what should be the factor for converting this volume from ATPS to BTPS (Appendix F)? What is the corrected V_T under BTPS conditions?

(A) 1.080; 540 mL
(B) 1.080; 580 mL
(C) 1.075; 624 mL
(D) 1.075; 780 mL

7d. A gas volume measured at room temperature (e.g., 25°C) is:

(A) greater than the volume at body temperature.
(B) greater than the volume at any temperature.
(C) lower than the volume at body temperature.
(D) lower than the volume at any temperature.

Chapter

8

Bicarbonate Corrections of Base Deficit

This equation calculates the amount of sodium bicarbonate needed to correct severe metabolic acidosis. The value $\frac{1}{4}$ in the equation represents the amount of extracellular water in the body.

During cardiopulmonary resuscitation or when the patient's perfusion is unsatisfactory, the entire calculated amount is given.

If cardiac massage is not required, half of the calculated dose is given initially to prevent overcompensation. Bicarbonate may not be needed when the arterial pH is greater than 7.20 or the base deficit is less than 10 mEq/L. For patients with diabetic ketoacidosis, bicarbonate may best be withheld until the pH is less than 7.10.

According to the *Textbook of Advanced Cardiac Life Support* by AHA, use of bicarbonate in cardiopulmonary resuscitation is not recommended. However, in sever, pre-existing metabolic acidosis, 1 mEq/kg of sodium bicarbonate may be used; subsequent doses should not exceed 33% to 50% of the calculated bicarbonate requirement. Refer to the current *ACLS* guidelines for specific indications.

EQUATION

$$HCO_3^- = \frac{(BD \times kg)}{4}$$

HCO_3^- : Sodium bicarbonate needed to correct severe base deficit, in mEq/L

BD : Base deficit in mEq/L, negative base excess $(-BE)$ determined by arterial blood gases

kg : Body weight in kilograms

EXAMPLE

How many mEq/L of bicarbonate are needed to correct a base deficit of 12 mEq/L if the patient's body weight is 60 kg? If the initial dose is $\frac{1}{2}$ of the calculated amount, what is the initial dose?

$$HCO_3^- = \frac{(BD \times kg)}{4}$$

$$= \frac{(12 \times 60)}{4}$$

$$= \frac{(720)}{4}$$

$$= 180 \text{ mEq/L}$$

Initial dose $= \frac{1}{2} \times 180$ or 90 mEq/L

EXERCISE

Calculate the amount of bicarbonate for a 70-kg patient whose BE is -18 mEq/L. What is the initial dose?

[Answer: $HCO_3^- = 315$ mEq/L; initial dose = 158 mEq/L]

REFERENCES

medscape.com (6/17/2010); Shapiro (1)

SELF-ASSESSMENT QUESTIONS

8a. A 53-kg patient has a base deficit of 30 mEq/L. If indicated, the initial amount of bicarbonate needed for this patient is about:

(A) Bicarbonate is not indicated.
(B) 265 mEq/L.
(C) 199 mEq/L.
(D) 133 mEq/L.

8b. Calculate the amount of bicarbonate needed to correct a base deficit of 20 mEq/L for a patient weighing 80 kg. If the initial dose is 1/2 of the calculated amount, what should be the initial dose?

(A) 800 mEq/L; initial dose = 400 mEq/L
(B) 400 mEq/L; initial dose = 200 mEq/L
(C) 200 mEq/L; initial dose = 100 mEq/L
(D) 80 mEq/L; initial dose = 40 mEq/L

8c. How much bicarbonate is needed to correct a base deficit of 16 mEq/L for a patient whose body weight is 70 kg? What should be the initial dose if half of the calculated amount is needed?

(A) 16 mEq/L; initial dose = 8 mEq/L
(B) 150 mEq/L; initial dose = 75 mEq/L
(C) 180 mEq/L; initial dose = 90 mEq/L
(D) 280 mEq/L; initial dose = 140 mEq/L

8d. The base deficit (− base excess) can be determined by:

(A) arterial blood gases.
(B) body weight in lb.
(C) body weight in kg.
(D) serum bicarbonate.

Chapter

9

Body Surface Area

NOTES

The body surface area (*BSA*) is used to calculate the cardiac index, the stroke volume index, or the drug dosages for adults and children. One way to find the body surface area is to use the DuBois Body Surface Chart (Appendix I). If the chart is not available, this BSA equation can be used.

To use the equation, the patient's body weight in *kilograms* must be known. Divide the body weight in pounds by 2.2 to get kilograms.

EQUATION 1

$$BSA = \frac{(4 \times kg) + 7}{kg + 90}$$

BSA : Body surface area in m^2
kg   : Body weight in kilograms

EQUATION 2

$$BSA = 0.04950 \times kg^{0.6046}$$
(This formula requires a calculator with power function.)

NORMAL VALUE

Adult average $BSA = 1.7 \text{ m}^2$

EXAMPLE

What is the calculated body surface area of a child weighing 44 pounds?

$$44 \text{ lbs} = \frac{44}{2.2} \text{ kg}$$
$$= 20 \text{ kg}$$

$$BSA = \frac{(4 \times kg) + 7}{kg + 90}$$
$$= \frac{(4 \times 20) + 7}{20 + 90}$$
$$= \frac{80 + 7}{110}$$
$$= \frac{87}{110}$$
$$= 0.79 \text{ m}^2$$

EXERCISE 1

Calculate the body surface area of a 132-lb patient.

[Answer: $BSA = 1.65 \text{ m}^2$]

EXERCISE 2

Use the DuBois Body Surface Chart in Appendix I to find the body surface area of a person who is 5′6″ and 140 lb. Using the equation and weight provided, calculate the body surface area.

[Answer: *BSA* (chart) = 1.72 m^2; *BSA* (calculated) = 1.70 m^2]

REFERENCE   Wilkins (1)

SEE   *Appendix I, DuBois Body Surface Chart*

SELF-ASSESSMENT QUESTIONS

9a. Calculate the body surface area (BSA) of a person weighing 80 kg.

Given: $BSA = \dfrac{(4 \times kg) + 7}{kg + 90}$.

(A) 3.14 m

(B) 1.92 m

(C) 1.92 m^2

(D) 3.14 m^2

9b. What is the calculated body surface area (BSA) of a person weighing 120 lb? (2.2 lb = 1 kg.) If the same person is 5′5″ tall, what is the body surface area using the DuBois Body Surface Chart (Appendix I)?

(A) 1.56 m^2; 1.59 m^2

(B) 1.76 m^2; 1.59 m^2

(C) 1.89 m^2; 1.66 m^2

(D) 1.93 m^2; 1.66 m^2

9c. To use the DuBois Body Surface Chart, the following must be known:

(A) weight and height.

(B) weight.

(C) height.

(D) age and weight.

Chapter

10

Cardiac Index (*CI*)

NOTES

Normal cardiac output for a resting adult ranges from 4 to 8 L/min.

Cardiac index (*CI*) is used to normalize cardiac output measurements among patients of varying body sizes. For instance, a cardiac output of 4 L/min may be normal for an average-sized person but low for a large-sized person. The cardiac index will be able to distinguish this difference based on body size.

CI values between 1.8 and 2.5 L/min/m^2 indicate hypoperfusion. Values less than 1.8 may be indicative of cardiogenic shock.

EQUATION

$$CI = \frac{CO}{BSA}$$

CI : Cardiac index in L/min/m^2
CO : Cardiac output in L/min (Q_T)
BSA : Body surface area in m^2

NORMAL VALUE

2.5 to 3.5 L/min/m^2

EXAMPLE

Given: Cardiac output = 4 L/min
       Body surface area = 1.4 m^2
Calculate the cardiac index.

$$CI = \frac{CO}{BSA}$$

$$= \frac{4}{1.4}$$

$$- 2.86 \text{ L/min/m}^2$$

EXERCISE

Given: Cardiac output = 4 L/min
       Body surface area = 2.5 m^2
Find the cardiac index (*CI*).

[Answer: *CI* = 1.6 L/min/m^2]

REFERENCES

Des Jardins; Wilkins (2)

SEE

Appendix I, DuBois Body Surface Chart; Appendix Q, Hemodynamic Normal Ranges.

SELF-ASSESSMENT QUESTIONS

10a. Given: Cardiac output = 4.5 L/min, body surface area = 1.0 m^2. What is the calculated cardiac index?

(A) 0.22 m^2/L/min

(B) 3.5 L/min/m^2

(C) 4.5 L/min/m^2

(D) 4.5 m^2/L/min

10b. Given the following measurements from a patient in the coronary intensive care unit: cardiac output = 5 L/min, body surface area = 1.7 m^2. What is the patient's cardiac index? Is it normal for this patient?

(A) 2.9 L/min/m^2; abnormal

(B) 2.9 L/min/m^2; normal

(C) 3.3 L/min/m^2; abnormal

(D) 3.3 L/min/m^2; normal

10c. An 85-kg patient has the following measurements: cardiac output = 5 L/min, body surface area = 2.9 m^2. What is the calculated cardiac index? Is it normal for this patient?

(A) 1.7 L/min/m^2; abnormal

(B) 1.7 L/min/m^2; normal

(C) 14.5 L/min/m^2; normal

(D) 14.5 L/min/m^2; abnormal

10d. The following measurements are obtained from a patient whose admitting diagnosis is Pickwickian syndrome with obstructive sleep apnea: cardiac output (*CO*) = 6 L/min, body surface area = 3.3 m^2. Is the patient's cardiac output within the normal range? Is the cardiac index (*CI*) normal?

(A) *CO* within normal range; *CI* abnormal

(B) *CO* and *CI* within normal range

(C) *CO* abnormal; *CI* within normal range

(D) *CO* and *CI* abnormal

10e. The following values are obtained from a 50-year-old patient with congestive heart failure: cardiac output = 3.0 L/min, body surface area = 1.0 m^2. Is the patient's cardiac output (*CO*) normal? Cardiac index (*CI*)?

(A) *CO* within normal range; *CI* abnormal

(B) *CO* and *CI* within normal range

(C) *CO* abnormal; *CI* within normal range

(D) *CO* and *CI* abnormal

10f. Ms. Morgan, a 68-year-old postsurgical patient, has a cardiac output of 4.9 L/min. If her estimated body surface area is 1.4 m^2, what is her cardiac index? Is it within the normal range?

(A) 3.5 L/min/m^2; normal

(B) 3.5 L/min/m^2; abnormal

(C) 4.1 L/min/m^2; normal

(D) 4.1 L/min/m^2; abnormal

Chapter

11

Cardiac Output (*CO*): Fick's Estimated Method

NOTES

The *CO* equation is used to calculate the cardiac output per minute.

The O_2 consumption ($130 \times BSA$) used in the equation is an estimate of the average oxygen consumption rate of an adult. This estimate is easier and faster to use than an actual measurement, but it may give inaccurate cardiac output determinations, particularly in patients with unusually high or low metabolic (O_2 consumption) rates.

Under normal conditions, the cardiac output is directly related to oxygen consumption (i.e., the cardiac output would increase in cases of increased oxygen consumption). If the cardiac output fails to keep up with the oxygen consumption needs, the $C(a-\bar{v})O_2$ increases.

EQUATION 1

$$CO = \frac{O_2 \text{ consumption}}{C_aO_2 - C_{\bar{v}}O_2}$$

EQUATION 2

$$CO = \frac{130 \times BSA}{C_aO_2 - C_{\bar{v}}O_2}$$

CO : Cardiac output in L/min (Q_T)

O_2 consumption: Estimated to be $130 \times BSA$, in mL/min ($\dot{V}O_2$)

C_aO_2 : Arterial oxygen content in vol%

: Mixed venous oxygen content in vol%

130 : Estimated O_2 consumption rate of an adult, in mL/min/m^2

BSA : Body surface area in m^2

NORMAL VALUE

CO = 4 to 8 L/min

EXAMPLE

Given: Body surface area = 1.6 m^2
Arterial O_2 content = 20 vol%
Mixed venous O_2 content = 15 vol%

$$CO = \frac{O_2 \text{ consumption}}{C_aO_2 - C_{\bar{v}}O_2}$$

$$= \frac{130 \times BSA}{C_aO_2 - C_{\bar{v}}O_2}$$

$$= \frac{130 \times 1.6}{20\% - 15\%}$$

$$= \frac{208}{5\%}$$

$$= \frac{208}{0.05}$$

$$= 4160 \text{ mL/min or } 4.16 \text{ L/min}$$

EXERCISE

Given: BSA = 1.2 m^2
C_aO_2 = 19 vol%
$C_{\bar{v}}O_2$ = 14 vol%

Calculate the cardiac output using Fick's estimated method.

[Answer: CO = 3,120 mL/min or 3.12 L/min]

REFERENCE

Wilkins (2)

SEE

Oxygen Consumption ($\dot{V}O_2$); Oxygen Content, Arterial (C_aO_2); Oxygen Content, Mixed Venous($C_{\bar{v}}O_2$); Appendix I, DuBois Body Surface Chart; Appendix Q, Hemodynamic Normal Ranges.

SELF-ASSESSMENT QUESTIONS

11a. Since oxygen consumption in mL/min can be estimated by using the formula 130 mL/min/m^2 × BSA m^2, what is the estimated O_2 consumption for a patient whose body surface area (BSA) is 1.5 m^2?

    (A) 100 mL/min
    (B) 130 mL/min
    (C) 150 mL/min
    (D) 195 mL/min

11b. Given: oxygen consumption ($\dot{V}O_2$) = 156 mL, arterial O_2 content (C_aO_2) = 19 vol%, mixed venous O_2 content ($C_{\bar{v}}O_2$) = 15 vol%. Calculate the cardiac output using Fick's estimated method.

    (A) 156 mL/min
    (B) 892 mL/min
    (C) 2.3 L/min
    (D) 3.9 L/min

11c. The following hemodynamic values are obtained from a patient in the intensive care unit: estimated oxygen consumption ($\dot{V}O_2$) = 180 mL, arterial O_2 content (C_aO_2) = 18.4 vol%, mixed venous O_2 content ($C_{\bar{v}}O_2$) = 14.4 vol%. Calculate the cardiac output using Fick's estimated method. Is it normal?

    (A) 4.5 L/min; normal
    (B) 5.5 L/min; normal
    (C) 6 L/min; abnormal
    (D) 6.5 L/min; abnormal

11d. A patient whose body surface area is about 1.4 m^2 has the following oxygen content values: C_aO_2 = 19.5 vol%, $C_{\bar{v}}O_2$ = 14.5 vol%. What is the cardiac output based on Fick's estimated method?

    (A) 2.73 L/min
    (B) 2.98 L/min
    (C) 3.64 L/min
    (D) 4.52 L/min

Chapter

12

Cerebral Perfusion Pressure

NOTES

To calculate the CPP, the MAP and ICP must have the same unit of measurement (mm Hg). The MAP may be obtained directly from the monitor of an indwelling arterial catheter. MAP may also be calculated from the indirect blood pressure measurements:

MAP = (systolic BP + 2 × diastolic BP) / 3

The ICP is obtained directly from the intracranial pressure monitor.

The CPP has a normal limit of 70 to 80 mm Hg. Low CPP indicates that the cerebral perfusion is inadequate and it is associated with a high mortality rate. There is no class I evidence for the optimum level of CPP, but the critical threshold is believed to be from 70 to 80 mm Hg. Mortality increased about 20% for each 10 mm Hg drop in CPP. In studies involving severe head injuries, 35% reduction in mortality was achieved when the CPP was maintained above 70 mm Hg.

Since CPP is the difference between MAP and ICP, changes in MAP or ICP will directly affect the CPP. A higher CPP can be achieved by raising the MAP or lowering the ICP. In the absence of hemorrhage, the MAP should be managed initially by fluid balance, followed by a vasopressor such as norepinephrine or dopamine. Systemic hypotension (SBP < 90 mm Hg) should be avoided and controlled as soon as possible because early hypotension is associated with

EQUATION

CPP = MAP − ICP

CPP : Cerebral Perfusion Pressure
MAP : Mean Arterial Pressure
ICP : Intracranial Pressure

NORMAL VALUE

70 to 80 mm Hg

EXAMPLE 1

Calculate the CPP given the following data: MAP = 90 mm Hg, ICP = 14 mm Hg. Is the calculated CCP within normal limits?

CPP = MAP − ICP
    = 90 mm Hg − 14 mm Hg
    = 76 mm Hg

CPP is within normal limit of 70 to 80 mm Hg.

EXAMPLE 2

The arterial blood pressure of a patient is 110/60 mm Hg. The ICP measured at the same time is 18 mm Hg. Is the calculated CCP normal?

MAP = (systolic BP + 2 × diastolic BP) / 3
    = (110 + 2 × 60) / 3
    = (110 + 120) / 3
    = 230 / 3
    = 76.66 or 77 mm Hg

CPP = MAP − ICP
    = 77 mm Hg − 18 mm Hg
    = 59 mm Hg

CPP is lower than normal limit of 70 to 80 mm Hg.

EXERCISE 1

Given: MAP = 110 mm Hg, ICP = 22 mm Hg. Calculate the CCP. Is it within the normal limit?

[Answer: CPP = 88 mm Hg; higher than normal limit of 70 to 80 mm Hg]

NOTES (continued)
increased morbidity and
mortality following severe
brain injury.

The ICP for normal subjects
is 8 to 12 mm Hg. In practice,
the ICP is usually maintained
within clinical normal limits
(i.e., < 20 mm Hg).

EXERCISE 2

A patient has a mean arterial pressure of 90 mm Hg and
an intracranial pressure (ICP) of 20 mm Hg. Calculate the
cerebral perfusion pressure (CPP). Is it normal?

[Answer: CPP = 70 mm Hg; within normal limit of
70 to 80 mm Hg]

REFERENCE

Chang

SELF-ASSESSMENT QUESTIONS

12a. Which of the following conditions is indicative of poor patient
outcome resulting from lack of perfusion to the brain?

(A) High arterial blood pressure
(B) Low cerebral perfusion pressure
(C) High mean arterial pressure
(D) Low intracranial pressure

12b. Calculate the cerebral perfusion pressure given the following
data: mean arterial pressure = 70 mm Hg, intracranial pressure
= 18 mm Hg. Is the calculated CCP within normal limits?

(A) 52 mm Hg; lower than normal limit
(B) 52 mm Hg; higher than normal limit
(C) 98 mm Hg; within normal limit
(D) 98 mm Hg; higher than normal limit

12c. The mean arterial pressure of a patient is 100 mm Hg. The
intracranial pressure is 22 mm Hg. What is the calculated cerebral
perfusion pressure? Is it normal?

(A) 78 mm Hg; abnormal
(B) 78 mm Hg; normal
(C) 122 mm Hg; abnormal
(D) 122 mm Hg; normal

12d. The arterial blood pressure of a patient is 90/50 mm Hg. The ICP
on the monitor shows 20 mm Hg. What is the calculated CPP? Is
it normal?

(A) 76 mm Hg; normal
(B) 66 mm Hg; normal
(C) 43 mm Hg; abnormal
(D) 53 mm Hg; abnormal

12e. A patient has an arterial blood pressure of 120/70 mm Hg and an
intracranial pressure of 28 mm Hg. What is the calculated CPP?
Is the CPP within the normal limit?

(A) 64 mm Hg; within normal limit of 60 to 70 mm Hg
(B) 64 mm Hg; lower than normal limit of 70 to 80 mm Hg
(C) 59 mm Hg; within normal limit of 50 to 60 mm Hg
(D) 59 mm Hg; lower than normal limit of 70 to 80 mm Hg

Chapter

13

Compliance: Dynamic (C_{dyn})

© Cengage Learning 2012

NOTES

Dynamic compliance is used to assess changes in the nonelastic (airway) resistance to air flow.

When the dynamic compliance changes *independently*, without corresponding change in static compliance, it is indicative of airway resistance changes. For example, if the dynamic compliance decreases with minimal or no decrease in static compliance, it is likely caused by an increase in nonelastic (airway) resistance. This type of resistance change may include bronchospasm, main-stem intubation, kinked tubing or endotracheal tube, mucus plugs, etc.

EQUATION

$$C_{dyn} = \frac{\Delta V}{\Delta P}$$

C_{dyn} : Dynamic compliance in mL/cm H_2O

ΔV : Corrected tidal volume in mL

ΔP : Pressure change (Peak inspiratory pressure – *PEEP*) in cm H_2O

NORMAL VALUE

30 to 40 mL/cm H_2O
If the patient is intubated, use serial measurements to establish trend.

EXAMPLE

Given: ΔV = 500 mL
Peak inspiratory pressure = 30 cm H_2O
PEEP = 10 cm H_2O
Calculate the dynamic compliance.

$$C_{dyn} = \frac{\Delta V}{\Delta P}$$

$$= \frac{500}{30 - 10}$$

$$= \frac{500}{20}$$

$$= 25 \text{ mL/cm } H_2O$$

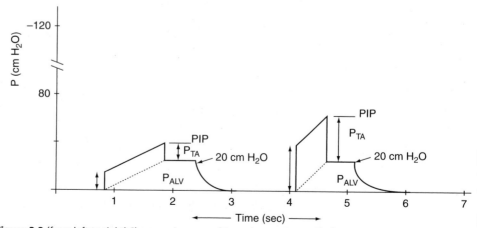

Figure 2-2 (from left to right) Shows an increase of transairway pressure (P_{TA}). Airway resistance is increased because the PIP is increased while the P_{ALV} (lung compliance) remains unchanged.

EXERCISE

Given: Corrected tidal volume   = 600 mL
       Peak inspiratory pressure = 40 cm H_2O
       PEEP   = 5 cm H_2O

Calculate the dynamic compliance.

[Answer: C_{dyn} = 17.1 or 17 mL/cm H_2O]

REFERENCES

Chang; Kacmarek

SEE

Corrected Tidal Volume (V_T); Compliance: Static (C_{st}).

SELF-ASSESSMENT QUESTIONS

13a. Given: corrected tidal volume = 650 mL, peak airway pressure = 32 cm H_2O. Calculate the dynamic compliance.

   (A) 10 mL/cm H_2O
   (B) 15 mL/cm H_2O
   (C) 20 mL/cm H_2O
   (D) 25 mL/cm H_2O

13b. What is the patient's dynamic compliance if the corrected tidal volume = 600 mL, peak airway pressure = 45 cm H_2O, and *PEEP* = 15 cm H_2O?

   (A) 13 mL/cm H_2O
   (B) 20 mL/cm H_2O
   (C) 26 mL/cm H_2O
   (D) 41 mL/cm H_2O

13c. A mechanically ventilated patient has the following measurements: corrected tidal volume = 700 mL, peak airway pressure = 45 cm H_2O, plateau pressure = 35 cm H_2O, and *PEEP* = 10 cm H_2O. What is the dynamic compliance?

   (A) 28 mL/cm H_2O
   (B) 24 mL/cm H_2O
   (C) 20 mL/cm H_2O
   (D) 15 mL/cm H_2O

13d. If a patient's corrected tidal volume is 500 mL and the corresponding peak airway pressure is 20 cm H_2O, what is the calculated dynamic compliance?

   (A) 16 mL/cm H_2O
   (B) 20 mL/cm H_2O
   (C) 25 mL/cm H_2O
   (D) 40 mL/cm H_2O

Chapter

14

Compliance: Static (C_{st})

NOTES

Static compliance is used to assess changes of the elastic (lung parenchymal) resistance to air flow.

The static compliance causes the dynamic compliance to increase or decrease correspondingly, and by similar proportion.

When the static and dynamic compliances decrease in the same proportion, it is indicative of an increase of elastic (lung parenchymal) resistance such as pneumonia or pulmonary edema. On the other hand, improvement of any lung parenchymal disease would increase the static *and* dynamic compliance.

EQUATION

$$C_{st} = \frac{\Delta V}{\Delta P}$$

C_{st} : Static compliance in mL/cm H_2O
ΔV : Corrected tidal volume in mL
ΔP : Pressure change (Plateau pressure – *PEEP*) in cm H_2O

NORMAL VALUE

40 to 60 mL/cm H_2O
If the patient is intubated, use serial measurements to establish trend.

EXAMPLE

Given: ΔV = 500 mL
Plateau pressure = 20 cm H_2O
PEEP = 5 cm H_2O
Calculate the static compliance:

$$C_{st} = \frac{\Delta V}{\Delta P}$$

$$= \frac{500}{20 - 5}$$

$$= \frac{500}{15}$$

$$= 33.3 \text{ or } 33 \text{ mL/cm } H_2O$$

EXERCISE

Given: Corrected tidal volume = 600 mL
Plateau pressure = 25 cm H_2O
PEEP = 5 cm H_2O
Calculate the static compliance.

[Answer: C_{st} = 30 mL/cm H_2O]

REFERENCES

Chang; Kacmarek

SEE

Corrected Tidal Volume (V_T); Compliance: Dynamic (C_{dyn}).

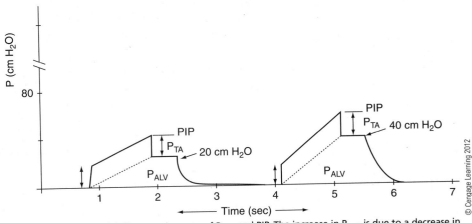

Figure 2-3 (from left to right) Shows an increase of P_{ALV} and PIP. The increase in P_{ALV} is due to a decrease in lung compliance. The increase in PIP is due to an increase of the P_{ALV} (plateau pressure). Airway resistance is unchanged because the P_{TA} measurements remain unchanged.

SELF-ASSESSMENT QUESTIONS

14a. $\dfrac{\textit{Corrected tidal volume}}{\textit{plateau pressure}}$ is equal to :

    (A) static compliance

    (B) dynamic compliance

    (C) airway resistance

    (D) airway conductance

14b. Given the following ventilation parameters, corrected tidal volume = 700 mL, plateau pressure = 30 cm H_2O, calculate the static compliance.

    (A) 7 mL/cm H_2O

    (B) 10 mL/cm H_2O

    (C) 20.8 mL/cm H_2O

    (D) 23.3 mL/cm H_2O

14c. Calculate a patient's static compliance given the following data: corrected tidal volume = 650 mL, plateau pressure = 30 cm H_2O, and *PEEP* = 10 cm H_2O.

    (A) 43.7 mL/cm H_2O

    (B) 32.5 mL/cm H_2O

    (C) 21.6 mL/cm H_2O

    (D) 18.2 mL/cm H_2O

14d. The following measurements are obtained from a patient who is on a ventilator: corrected tidal volume = 780 mL, peak airway pressure = 55 cm H_2O, plateau pressure = 35 cm H_2O, and *PEEP* = 10 cm H_2O. What is the static compliance?

    (A) 78 mL/cm H_2O

    (B) 31.2 mL/cm H_2O

    (C) 22.3 mL/cm H_2O

    (D) 17.3 mL/cm H_2O

14e. Four sets of values have been obtained to determine the optimum *PEEP*, based on the best static compliance. Which of the following measurements indicates the best static compliance?

	Corrected Tidal Volume	Plateau Pressure	*PEEP*
(A)	750 mL	32 cm H_2O	8 cm H_2O
(B)	750 mL	34 cm H_2O	10 cm H_2O
(C)	700 mL	32 cm H_2O	12 cm H_2O
(D)	700 mL	36 cm H_2O	14 cm H_2O

Chapter
15
Compliance: Total (C_T)

EQUATION

$$\frac{1}{C_T} = \frac{1}{C_L} + \frac{1}{C_{cw}}$$

$\dfrac{1}{C_T}$: Reciprocal of total compliance (lung and chest wall)

$\dfrac{1}{C_L}$: Reciprocal of lung compliance

$\dfrac{1}{C_{cw}}$: Reciprocal of chest-wall compliance

This equation describes the relationship among total compliance, lung compliance, and chest-wall compliance. It is essential to note that the *reciprocals* of these values are related. For example, if the lung and chest-wall compliance values are both 0.2 L/cm H_2O, the sum of these two reciprocals (total compliance) is 0.1 L/cm H_2O.

$$\frac{1}{0.2} + \frac{1}{0.2} = \frac{(1+1)}{0.2}$$
$$= \frac{2}{0.2}$$
$$= \frac{1}{0.1}$$

With an intact lung-thorax system, the lung compliance equals the chest-wall compliance. When this condition exists, the total compliance is half of the lung compliance or chest-wall compliance.

REFERENCE

Wojciechowski

SELF-ASSESSMENT QUESTIONS

15a. Which of the following groups of compliance values equal one
 another in an intact lung-thorax system?

 (A) Lung compliance and chest-wall compliance
 (B) Total compliance and chest-wall compliance
 (C) Total compliance and lung compliance
 (D) Total compliance, lung compliance, and chest-wall
  compliance

15b. Total compliance is about _____ L/cm H_2O, _____ the
 normal lung compliance value.

 (A) 0.1; twice
 (B) 0.1; half of
 (C) 0.2; twice
 (D) 0.2; half of

15c. The normal chest-wall compliance is about _____ L/cm H_2O,
 _____ the normal lung compliance value.

 (A) 0.1; twice
 (B) 0.1; same as
 (C) 0.2; half of
 (D) 0.2; same as

15d. Under normal conditions, all of the following statements are true
 except:

 (A) Chest-wall compliance is same as lung compliance.
 (B) Chest-wall compliance is greater than total compliance.
 (C) Lung compliance is greater than total compliance.
 (D) The sum of lung and chest wall compliance is greater than
  total compliance.

Chapter

16
Corrected Tidal Volume (V_T)

NOTE

The tubing compression factor can be determined by the following procedures: (1) Set the frequency at 10 to 16/min and the tidal volume between 100 and 200 mL with minimum flow rate and maximum pressure limit; (2) completely occlude the patient Y-connection of the ventilator circuit; (3) record the observed expired volume (mL) and the peak inspiratory pressure (cm H_2O); and (4) divide the observed expired volume by the peak inspiratory pressure. The result is the tubing compression factor in mL/cm H_2O.

EQUATION

Corrected V_T = Expired V_T – Tubing Volume

Expired V_T : Expired tidal volume in mL
Tubing volume : Volume "lost" in tubing during inspiratory phase (Pressure change × 3 mL/cm H_2O)*

EXAMPLE

Expired V_T = 650 mL
Peak inspiratory pressure = 25 cm H_2O
Positive end-expiratory pressure (*PEEP*) = 5 cm H_2O
Tubing compression factor = 3 mL/cm H_2O*

Calculate the corrected tidal volume.

Tubing volume = Pressure change × 3 mL/cm H_2O
= (25 − 5) cm H_2O × 3 mL/cm H_2O
= 20 × 3 mL
= 60 mL

Corrected V_T = Expired V_T − Tubing volume
= 650 − 60
= 590 mL

EXERCISE

Expired V_T = 780 mL
Peak inspiratory pressure = 45 cm H_2O
PEEP = 10 cm H_2O
Tubing compression factor = 3 mL/cm H_2O

Calculate the corrected tidal volume.

[Answer: Corrected V_T = 675 mL]

REFERENCE

Wilkins (2)

*The tubing compression factor ranges from 1 to 8 mL/cm H_2O.
This factor may change according to (1) the type of ventilator used, (2) the type of circuit used, and (3) the water level in the humidifier.*

SELF-ASSESSMENT QUESTIONS

16a. What is the tubing compression volume if the tubing compression factor is 3 mL/cm H_2O and the pressure change is 30 cm H_2O?

(A) 30 mL

(B) 33 mL

(C) 60 mL

(D) 90 mL

16b. The information below is obtained from a routine ventilator check. Calculate the corrected tidal volume.

$$\text{Expired } V_T = 700 \text{ mL}$$
$$\text{Peak inspiratory pressure} = 45 \text{ cm } H_2O$$
$$PEEP = 5 \text{ cm } H_2O$$
$$\text{Tubing compression factor} = 3 \text{ mL/cm } H_2O$$

(A) 565 mL

(B) 660 mL

(C) 600 mL

(D) 580 mL

16c. Calculate the corrected tidal volume with the following information obtained during a ventilator check:

$$\text{Expired } V_T = 780 \text{ mL}$$
$$\text{Peak inspiratory pressure} = 45 \text{ cm } H_2O$$
$$PEEP = 5 \text{ cm } H_2O$$
$$\text{Tubing compression factor} = 5 \text{ mL/cm } H_2O$$

(A) 555 mL

(B) 580 mL

(C) 620 mL

(D) 755 mL

Chapter

17

Correction Factor

NOTES
Example 1

In this example, the expected pressure is the barometric pressure, 1,000 cm H_2O or 735 mm Hg. During inspiration, the circuit pressure is 50 cm H_2O higher than the barometric pressure. The measured pressure is therefore 1,050 cm H_2O (1,000 + 50). The correction factor 0.952 is used to multiply the F_IO_2 as recorded by the analyzer. For example, if the oxygen analyzer reads 60%, the corrected F_IO_2 becomes 57% (60% $\times$ 0.952 = 57.12%).

Example 2

In the first part of Example 2, the measured volume is greater than the expected volume during calibration. The correction factor is therefore less than 1. Once a "correction" factor is obtained, subsequent measurements may be "corrected" by multiplying them by this correction factor. For example, if the correction factor is 0.993 and the spirometer reads a tidal volume of 600 mL, the corrected tidal volume becomes 596 mL (600 $\times$ 0.993 = 595.8 mL).

In the second part of Example 2, the measured volume is smaller than the expected volume during calibration. The correction factor is therefore greater than 1. For example, if the correction factor is 1.014 and the spirometer reads a tidal volume of 600 mL, the corrected tidal volume becomes 608 mL (600 $\times$ 1.014 = 608.4 mL).

EQUATION

$$\text{Correction Factor} = \frac{\text{Expected}}{\text{Measured}}$$

Expected : Expected (input) measurements such as barometric pressure, volume in calibration syringe

Measured : Actual (output) measurements such as pressure in ventilator circuit, volume recorded by spirometry

NORMAL VALUE

Correction factor > 1 if expected > measured.
Correction factor not needed if expected = measured.
Corrected factor < 1 if expected < measured.

EXAMPLE 1

A galvanic cell oxygen analyzer is being used in a ventilator circuit (circuit pressure = 50 cm H_2O). If barometric pressure is 735 mm Hg (1,000 cm H_2O), what should be the correction factor for subsequent F_IO_2 measurements?

$$\begin{aligned}
\text{Correction factor} &= \frac{\text{Expected}}{\text{Measure}} \\
&= \frac{1000}{1000 + 50} \\
&= \frac{1000}{1050} \\
&= 0.952
\end{aligned}$$

EXAMPLE 2

A 3-L calibration syringe is used to calibrate the pulmonary function spirometer. If the spirometer records a volume of 3.02 L, what should be the correction factor for subsequent volume measurements?

$$\begin{aligned}
\text{Correction factor} &= \frac{\text{Expected}}{\text{Measured}} \\
&= \frac{3.00}{3.02} \\
&= 0.993
\end{aligned}$$

What should be the correction factor if the spirometer records a volume of 2.96 L?

$$\text{Correction factor} = \frac{\text{Expected}}{\text{Measured}}$$
$$= \frac{3.00}{2.96}$$
$$= 1.014$$

EXERCISE 1

A polarographic oxygen analyzer is being used in a ventilator circuit (circuit pressure = 45 cm H_2O). If barometric pressure is 996 cm H_2O, what should be the correction factor for all subsequent F_IO_2 measurements?

[Answer: Correction factor = 0.957]

EXERCISE 2

A 3-L calibration syringe is used to calibrate the pulmonary function spirometer. If the spirometer records a volume of 2.88 L, what should be the correction factor for subsequent volume measurements?

[Answer: Correction factor = 1.042]

What should be the correction factor if the spirometer records a volume of 3.07 L?

[Answer: Correction factor = 0.977]

REFERENCE

Ruppel

SEE

Pressure Conversions in Appendix BB to convert pressures from mm Hg to cm H_2O.

SELF-ASSESSMENT QUESTIONS

17a. The correction factor used in calibration of a pulmonary function spirometer or other similar device can be calculated by using the following solution:

(A) Expected value + Actual value
(B) Expected value – Actual value
(C) Expected value × Actual value
(D) $\dfrac{\text{Expected value}}{\text{Actual value}}$

17b. Exactly 3 L of air from a calibration syringe is used to calibrate the pulmonary function spirometer. The recorded volume is 2.89 L. Calculate the correction factor for subsequent volume measurements made by this spirometer.

(A) 0.926
(B) 0.963
(C) 1.038
(D) 1.045

17c. A known flow rate at precisely 4 L/sec is introduced into the spirometer, and the spirometer records a flow rate of 4.07 L/sec. What should be the correction factor for subsequent flow rate measurements?

(A) 1.017
(B) 0.953
(C) 0.970
(D) 0.983

17d. If the correction factor for a spirometer is 0.993 and the spirometer measures a vital capacity of 3.8 L, what should be the corrected vital capacity?

(A) 3.51 L
(B) 3.62 L
(C) 3.77 L
(D) 3.83 L

17e. A polarographic oxygen analyzer is being used in a ventilator circuit (circuit pressure = 45 cm H_2O). If barometric pressure is 900 cm H_2O, what should be the correction factor for all subsequent F_IO_2 measurements?

(A) 1.05
(B) 0.921
(C) 0.934
(D) 0.952

17f. A pressure-sensitive oxygen analyzer (galvanic cell) is used to measure the F_IO_2 in a ventilator circuit. Calculate the correction factor for the F_IO_2 measurements if the barometric pressure is 1,003 cm H_2O and the circuit pressure is 60 cm H_2O over the barometric pressure.

(A) 0.911
(B) 0.944
(C) 0.965
(D) 1.059

17g. The sensor of a galvanic cell oxygen analyzer is placed in-line of a ventilator circuit. An F_IO_2 reading of 60% is obtained. What is the corrected F_IO_2 if the correction factor is 0.934 for this oxygen analyzer?

(A) 56%
(B) 60%
(C) 62%
(D) 64%

Chapter

18

Dalton's Law of Partial Pressure

NOTES

Dalton's law, named for the English chemist John Dalton (1766–1844), states that the total pressure exerted by a gas mixture is equal to the sum of the partial pressures of all gases in the mixture. Water vapor is considered a gas, and it exerts water vapor pressure. Table 2-3 shows the gases that compose the barometric pressure in the absence of water vapor.

In unusual atmospheric environments, individual gas pressures increase in hyperbaric conditions (e.g., hyperbaric chamber, under water) and decrease in hypobaric conditions (e.g., high altitude) according to the percentage of the total volume each gas occupies.

EQUATION

Total pressure $= P_1 + P_2 + P_3 + ...$
Total pressure : Pressure of all gases in mixture
P_1 : Pressure of gas 1 in gas mixture
P_2 : Pressure of gas 2 in gas mixture
P_3 : Pressure of gas 3 in gas mixture
... : Pressure of other gases

TABLE 2-3 Gases That Compose the Barometric Pressure

GAS	%OF ATMOSPHERE	Partial Pressure of Dry Gas (mm Hg)
Nitrogen (N_2)	78.08	593
Oxygen (O_2)	20.95	159
Argon (Ar)	0.93	7
Carbon Dioxide (CO_2)	0.03	0.2

From Des Jardins, T.R., *Cardiopulmonary Anatomy and Physiology: Essentials of Respiratory Care,* 5th ed. Clifton Park, NY: Delmar Cengage Learning, 2008.

REFERENCES   Des Jardins; Wilkins (2)

SEE   *Partial Pressure of a Dry Gas.*

SELF-ASSESSMENT QUESTIONS

18a. The sum of partial pressures exerted by all gases in the atmosphere equals the barometric pressure. This is a statement of:

(A) Dalton's law.
(B) Henry's law.
(C) Charles' law.
(D) Graham's law.

18b. If the PO_2 is 100 mm Hg at one barometric pressure
(760 mm Hg), what is the approximate PO_2 if the pressure is
increased to 1,520 mm Hg in a hyperbaric chamber?

(A) 25 mm Hg
(B) 50 mm Hg
(C) 100 mm Hg
(D) 200 mm Hg

18c. The normal predicted PO_2 in an area 10,000 ft above sea level
should be _____ the PO_2 at sea level because of the _____
condition at high altitude.

(A) higher than; hyperbaric
(B) higher than; hypobaric
(C) lower than; hyperbaric
(D) lower than; hypobaric

18d. The most abundant gas in the atmosphere is:

(A) helium.
(B) oxygen.
(C) nitrogen.
(D) carbon dioxide.

Chapter

19

Deadspace to Tidal Volume Ratio (V_D/V_T)

NOTES

$\frac{V_D}{V_T}$ ratio is used to approximate the portion of tidal volume not taking part in gas exchange (i.e., wasted ventilation). A large $\frac{V_D}{V_T}$ ratio indicates ventilation is in excess of perfusion. Emphysema, positive-pressure ventilation, pulmonary embolism, and hypotension are some causes of increased deadspace ventilation.

For patients receiving mechanical ventilation, $\frac{V_D}{V_T}$ ratio of up to 60% is considered acceptable. This value is consistent with a normal $\frac{V_D}{V_T}$ after the patient is weaned off mechanical ventilation and extubated.

EQUATION

$$\frac{V_D}{V_T} = \frac{\left(P_aCO_2 - P_{\bar{E}}CO_2\right)}{P_aCO_2}$$

$\frac{V_D}{V_T}$: Deadspace to tidal volume ratio in %

P_aCO_2 : Arterial carbon dioxide tension in mm Hg

$P_{\bar{E}}CO_2$: Mixed expired carbon dioxide tension in mm Hg*

NORMAL VALUE

20 to 40% in patients breathing spontaneously
40 to 60% in patients receiving mechanical ventilation

EXAMPLE

Given: P_aCO_2 = 40 mm Hg
$P_{\bar{E}}CO_2$ = 30 mm Hg

Calculate the $\frac{V_D}{V_T}$ ratio.

$$\frac{V_D}{V_T} = \frac{\left(P_aCO_2 - P_{\bar{E}}CO_2\right)}{P_aCO_2}$$

$$= \frac{40 - 30}{40}$$

$$= \frac{10}{40}$$

$$= 0.25 \text{ or } 25\%$$

*$P_{\bar{E}}CO_2$ is measured by analyzing the PCO_2 of a sample of expired gas collected on the exhalation port of the ventilator circuit or via a one-way valve for spontaneously breathing patients. A 5-L bag can be used for sample collection. To prevent contamination of the gas sample, sigh breaths should not be included in this sample and exhaled gas should be completely isolated from the patient circuit. The P_aCO_2 is measured by analyzing an arterial blood gas sample obtained while collecting the exhaled gas sample.

EXERCISE

Given: P_aCO_2 = 30 mm Hg

$P_{\overline{E}}CO_2$ = 15 mm Hg

Calculate the $\dfrac{V_D}{V_T}$ ratio.

[Answer: $\dfrac{V_D}{V_T}$ = 0.50 or 50%]

REFERENCE Wilkins (2)

SELF-ASSESSMENT QUESTIONS

19a. A mixed, expired gas sample for analysis of partial pressure of CO_2 is required for calculation of:

(A) I:E ratio.
(B) air entrainment ratio.
(C) V_D/V_T ratio.
(D) cardiac index.

19b. The deadspace to tidal volume ratio (V_D/V_T) requires measurements of:

I.   Arterial PCO_2.
II. Venous PCO_2.
III. Mixed expired PCO_2.
IV. Mixed expired PO_2.
(A) I, III only
(B) I, IV only
(C) II, III, IV only
(D) II, IV only

19c. For intubated patients who are being ventilated by a mechanical ventilator, it is acceptable to have a V_D/V_T ratio of up to:

(A) 30%.
(B) 40%.
(C) 50%.
(D) 60%.

19d. Given: P_aCO_2 = 35 mm Hg, $P_{\overline{E}}CO_2$ = 20 mm Hg, P_aO_2 = 80 mm Hg, pH = 7.45. What is the V_D/V_T ratio?
(A) 26%
(B) 31% $\dfrac{35 - 20}{35} =$
(C) 35%
(D) 43%

19e. Given: P_aCO_2 = 40 mm Hg, $P_{\overline{E}}CO_2$ = 30 mm Hg. Calculate the V_D/V_T ratio.
(A) 10% $\dfrac{40 - 30}{40}$
(B) 20%
(C) 25%
(D) 30%

19f. A 55-year-old man was admitted to the hospital for shortness of breath. The following results were obtained: P_aCO_2 = 50 mm Hg, $P_{\overline{E}}CO_2$ = 30 mm Hg. What is the calculated V_D/V_T ratio?

(A) 15%

(B) 20%

(C) 30%

(D) 40%

$$\frac{50-30}{50} = \frac{20}{50} = 40\%$$

19g. A patient who is on a mechanical ventilator has the following measurements: P_aCO_2=45 mm Hg, $P_{\overline{E}}CO_2$ = 25 mm Hg. What is the patient's deadspace to tidal volume ratio? Is it normal?

(A) 44%; normal

(B) 44%; abnormal

(C) 55%; normal

(D) 55%; abnormal

$$\frac{45-25}{45} = \frac{20}{45} = 44\%$$

Chapter

20
Density (*D*) of Gases

NOTE

The density of gas molecules is directly proportional to the molecular weights. In general, atoms and molecules having lower atomic numbers (smaller atomic weights) are lighter than those having higher atomic numbers. Atomic weight is also known as atomic mass.

EQUATION

$$D = \frac{gmw\,(\text{g})}{22.4\,(\text{L})}$$

D : Density of gas in g/L
gmw : Gram molecular weight in g*

EXAMPLE 1

Calculate the density of carbon dioxide (CO_2).

$$D = \frac{gmw\,(\text{g})}{22.4\,(\text{L})}$$

$$= \frac{\text{atomic weight of C} + (\text{atomic weight of O} \times 2)}{22.4}$$

$$= \frac{12 + (16 \times 2)}{22.4}$$

$$= \frac{12 + 32}{22.4}$$

$$= \frac{44}{22.4}$$

$$= 1.96 \text{ g/L}$$

EXAMPLE 2

Calculate the density of air (21% O_2, 78% N_2, 1% Ar).

$$D = \frac{gmw\,(\text{g})}{22.4\,(\text{L})}$$

$$= \frac{0.21 \times (\text{wt. of O} \times 2) + 0.78 \times (\text{wt. of N} \times 2) + 0.01 \times (\text{wt. of Ar})}{22.4}$$

$$= \frac{0.21 \times (16 \times 2) + 0.78 \times (14 \times 2) + 0.01 \times (40)}{22.4}$$

$$= \frac{0.21 \times 32 + 0.78 \times 28 + 0.01 \times 40}{22.4}$$

$$= \frac{6.72 + 21.84 + 0.4}{22.4}$$

$$= \frac{28.96}{22.4}$$

$$= 1.29 \text{ g/L}$$

*gmw = Atomic weight × Number of atoms per molecule.

EXERCISE 1	Use the Periodic Chart of Elements in Appendix Z and find the atomic weight and gram molecular weight (*gmw*) of oxygen (O_2).
	[Answer: Atomic weight of O = 16 g; *gmw* of O_2 = 32 g]
EXERCISE 2	What is the density (*D*) of oxygen (O_2)?
	[Answer: *D* = 1.429 g/L]
EXERCISE 3	Calculate the density of a gas mixture of 70% helium (He) and 30% oxygen (O_2).
	[Answer: *D* = 0.554 g/L]
REFERENCE	Wilkins (2)
SEE	*Appendix Z, Periodic Chart of Elements.*

SELF-ASSESSMENT QUESTIONS

20a. Calculate the density of nitrogen (N_2) if the atomic weight for nitrogen is 14.

   (A) 0.31 g/L
   (B) 0.63 g/L
   (C) 1.25 g/L
   (D) 2.5 g/L

20b. Given: atomic weight of helium = 4 g. What is its gas density?

   (A) 0.18 g/L
   (B) 1.8 g/L
   (C) 18 g/L
   (D) 4 g/L

20c. Calculate the density of carbon dioxide (CO_2) given that the atomic weights for carbon and oxygen are 12 and 16, respectively.

   (A) 1.48 g/L
   (B) 1.61 g/L
   (C) 1.75 g/L
   (D) 1.96 g/L

20d. Calculate the density of a helium/oxygen mixture (80% He, 20% O_2). The atomic weights for helium and oxygen are 4 and 16, respectively.

   (A) 0.43 g/L
   (B) 0.52 g/L
   (C) 0.68 g/L
   (D) 0.79 g/L

20e. Which of the following gas element/molecules is the most dense? N_2, CO, O_2, or CO_2? Calculate and report their densities. The molecular weights for N_2, CO, O_2, and CO_2 are 28, 28, 32, and 44, respectively.

(A) N_2: 1.25 g/L
(B) CO: 1.25 g/L
(C) O_2: 1.43 g/L
(D) CO_2: 1.96 g/L

Chapter

21

Dosage Calculation: Intravenous Solution Infusion Dosage

NOTE

The infusion dosage is usually in mg/min or mcg/min. The dosage in 1 mL must first be converted to the proper unit (mg or mcg) before using the equation (i.e., 1 g = 1,000 mg; 1 mg = 1,000 mcg).

EQUATION

$$\text{Infusion dosage} = \frac{\text{Infusion rate} \times \text{Dosage in 1 mL}}{60 \text{ drops/mL}}$$

Infusion dosage: Infusion dosage of intravenous (IV) solution, in mg/min or mcg/min

Infusion rate : Infusion rate of intravenous (IV) solution in drops/min

Dosage in 1 mL : Concentration of drug, in mg/mL or mcg/mL

60 drops/mL : Represents 60 IV drops in 1 mL

EXAMPLE 1

A 10-mL ampule of bretylium tosylate containing 500 mg of drug is mixed in 250 mL of D5W. If an infusion rate of 30 drops/min is being administered to the patient, what is the infusion dosage per minute? Since 500 mg/250 mL = 2 mg/mL, this is used in the example as dosage in 1 mL. (See Dosage Calculation: Percent (%) Solution.)

$$\text{Infusion dosage} = \frac{\text{Infusion rate} \times \text{Dosage in 1 mL}}{60 \text{ drops/mL}}$$

$$= \frac{30 \text{ drops/min} \times 2 \text{ mg/mL}}{60 \text{ drops/mL}}$$

$$= \frac{60 \text{ mg/min}}{60}$$

$$= 1 \text{ mg/min}$$

EXAMPLE 2

1 mg of isoproterenol is mixed with 250 mL of D5W. If an infusion rate of 30 drops/min is being administered to the patient, what is the infusion dosage in mcg per minute? Since 1 mg/250 mL = 1,000 mcg/250 mL = 4 mcg/mL, this is used in this example as dosage in 1 mL. (See Dosage Calculation: Percent (%) Solution.)

$$\text{Infusion dosage} = \frac{\text{Infusion rate} \times \text{Dosage in 1 mL}}{60 \text{ drops/mL}}$$

$$= \frac{30 \text{ drops/min} \times 4 \text{ mcg/mL}}{60 \text{ drops/mL}}$$

$$= \frac{120 \text{ mcg/min}}{60}$$

$$= 2 \text{ mcg/min}$$

EXERCISE 1   A 2-mL vial of procainamide containing 1 g of drug is mixed in 250 mL of D5W. If an infusion rate of 30 drops/min is being administered to the patient, what is the infusion dosage in mg per minute?

[Answer: Infusion dosage = 2 mg/min]

EXERCISE 2   50 mg of Nipride are mixed with 250 mL of D5W. If an infusion rate of 3 drops/min is being given to the patient, what is the infusion dosage in mcg per minute?

[Answer: Infusion dosage = 10 mcg/min]

REFERENCE   www.Dosagehelp.com

SEE   *Dosage Calculation: Percent (%) Solution; Dosage Calculation: Intravenous Solution Infusion Rate.*

SELF-ASSESSMENT QUESTIONS

21a. One gram of procainamide hydrochloride is mixed with 250 mL of D5W. If this mixture is given to a patient at an infusion rate of 15 drops/min, what is the infusion dosage in mg/min?

(A) 0.5 mg/min
(B) 1 mg/min
(C) 2 mg/min
(D) 2.5 mg/min

21b. 50 mg (50,000 mcg) of sodium nitroprusside are mixed with 250 mL of D5W. At an infusion rate of 6 drops/min, what is the infusion dosage in mcg/min?

(A) 5 mcg/min
(B) 10 mcg/min
(C) 15 mcg/min
(D) 20 mcg/min

21c. A 250-mL D5W solution contains 1 ampule (200 mg) of dopamine hydrochloride. If the patient is receiving this IV solution at a rate of 18 drops/min, what is the infusion dosage in mcg/min?

(A) 240 mcg/min
(B) 260 mcg/min
(C) 280 mcg/min
(D) 300 mcg/min

21d. 50 mg of nitroglycerin are mixed with 250 mL of D5W, and the mixture is running at an infusion rate of 3 drops/min. What is the infusion dosage in mcg/min?

(A) 5 mcg/min
(B) 10 mcg/min
(C) 15 mcg/min
(D) 20 mcg/min

Chapter

22

Dosage Calculation: Intravenous Solution Infusion Rate

NOTES

It is essential to use the proper units (mg or mcg) in the infusion dosage and dosage in 1 mL. To find dosage in 1 mL, 1 g is usually converted to 1,000 mg and 1 mg to 1,000 mcg.

If the infusion dosage is related to a patient's *body weight* (i.e., n mg/kg/min or n mcg/kg/min), multiply the n by the patient's body weight in kg and use the equation as shown in Example 2. For example, if the infusion dosage is 5 mcg/kg/min, an 80-kg patient would require an infusion dosage of 400 mcg/min (5 mcg/kg/min × 80 kg).

EQUATION

$$\text{Infusion rate} = \frac{60 \text{ drops/mL} \times \text{Infusion dosage}}{\text{dosage in 1 mL}}$$

Infusion rate : Infusion rate of intravenous (IV) solution in drops/min

60 drops/mL : Represents 60 IV drops in 1 mL

Infusion dosage : Infusion dosage of intravenous (IV) solution, in mg/min or mcg/min

Dosage in 1 mL : Concentration of drug, in mg/mL or mcg/mL

EXAMPLE 1

1 g of lidocaine is mixed with 250 mL of D5W. If an infusion dosage of 2 mg/min is desired, what should be the infusion rate in drops/min? Since 1 g/250 mL = 1,000 mg/250 mL = 4 mg/mL, this is used as dosage in 1 mL.

$$\text{Infusion rate} = \frac{60 \text{ drops/mL} \times \text{Infusion dosage}}{\text{Dosage in 1 mL}}$$

$$= \frac{60 \text{ drops/mL} \times 2 \text{ mg/min}}{4 \text{ mg/mL}}$$

$$= \frac{120 \text{ drops/mL} \times \text{mg/min}}{4 \text{ mg/mL}}$$

$$= 30 \text{ drops/min}$$

EXAMPLE 2

200 mg (1 amp) of dopamine is mixed with 250 mL of D5W. If an infusion dosage of 5 mcg/kg/min is desired, what should be the infusion rate in drops/min for a patient weighing 80 kg?

For an 80-kg patient, the infusion dosage of 5 mcg/kg/min would become 400 mcg/min (5 mcg/kg/min × 80 kg). Since 200 mg/250 mL = 200,000 mcg/250 mL = 800 mcg/mL, this is used as dosage in 1 mL.

$$\text{Infusion rate} = \frac{60 \text{ drops/mL} \times \text{Infusion dosage}}{\text{Dosage in 1 mL}}$$

$$= \frac{60 \text{ drops/mL} \times 400 \text{ mcg/min}}{800 \text{ mcg/mL}}$$

$$= \frac{24,000 \text{ drops/mL} \times \text{mcg/min}}{800 \text{ mcg/mL}}$$

$$= 30 \text{ drops/min}$$

EXERCISE 1   Two 10-mL ampules of bretylium tosylate containing 500 mg of drug in each ampule is mixed with 250 mL of D5W, for a total amount of 1,000 mg/250 mL. If an infusion dosage of 2 mg/min is desired, what should be the infusion rate in drops/min?

[Answer: Infusion rate = 30 drops/min]

EXERCISE 2   1 mg of epinephrine is mixed with 250 mL of D5W. If an infusion dosage of 1 mcg/min is desired, what should be the infusion rate in drops/min?

[Answer: Infusion rate = 15 drops/min]

REFERENCE   www.Dosagehelp.com

SEE   *Dosage Calculation: Percent (%) Solution; Dosage Calculation: Intravenous Solution Infusion Dosage.*

SELF-ASSESSMENT QUESTIONS

22a. One gram of lidocaine is mixed with 250 mL of D5W. At an infusion dosage of 1.6 mg/min intravenously, what should be the infusion rate in drops/min?

(A) 18 drops/min
(B) 20 drops/min
(C) 22 drops/min
(D) 24 drops/min

22b. Two grams of bretylium tosylate are mixed with 500 mL of D5W for intravenous use. If an infusion dosage of 2 mg/min is desired, find the infusion rate in drops/min.

(A) 8 drops/min
(B) 24 drops/min
(C) 30 drops/min
(D) 40 drops/min

22c. Find the infusion rate in drops/min when 1 mg of isoproterenol in 250 mL of D5W is used for an infusion dosage of 2 mcg/min.

(A) 15 drops/min
(B) 20 drops/min
(C) 25 drops/min
(D) 30 drops/min

22d. A10-mL ampule of bretylium tosylate containing 500 mg of drug is mixed with 250 mL of D5W. If an infusion dosage of 1 mg/min is desired, what should be the infusion rate in drops/min?

(A) 25 drops/min
(B) 30 drops/min
(C) 35 drops/min
(D) 40 drops/min

22e. A 250-mL D5W solution contains 1 mg of epinephrine. If an infusion dosage of 2 mcg/min is needed, what should be the infusion rate in drops/min?

(A) 5 drops/min

(B) 15 drops/min

(C) 30 drops/min

(D) 40 drops/min

Chapter

23

Dosage Calculation:
Percent (%) Solutions

NOTES

In Example 2, the volume calculated must be diluted with normal saline or other diluents before use. This applies to almost all respiratory care bronchodilator stock solutions.

Drug dosage calculation for unit dose is similar to that shown in the examples.

EQUATION 1

Dosage = Volume used × Concentration of original solution

EQUATION 2

$$\text{Volume} = \frac{\text{Dosage desired}}{\text{Concentration of original solution}}$$

EXAMPLE 1

How many mg of isoproterenol are in 0.5 mL of a 1:100 (1%) drug solution?

SOLUTION A. [This calculation gives the answer in g. It must be converted to mg.]

Dosage = Volume used × Concentration of original solution
= 0.5 × 1%
= 0.5 × 0.01
= 0.005 g (or 5 mg)

SOLUTION B. The 1:100 or 1% solution can be rewritten as follows:

$$1\% = \frac{1\ \text{g}}{100\ \text{mL}}$$

$$= \frac{1{,}000\ \text{mg}}{100\ \text{mL}}$$

$$= 10\ \text{mg/mL}$$

[This calculation gives the answer in mg.]

Dosage = Volume used × Concentration of original solution
= 0.5 mL × 1%
= 0.5 mL × 10 mg/mL
= 5 mg

EXAMPLE 2

An isoproterenol solution has a concentration of 1:200. How much volume is needed if 2.5 mg of the active ingredient is desired?

$$\text{Volume} = \frac{\text{Dosage desired}}{\text{Concentration of original solution}}$$

$$= \frac{2.5\ \text{mg}}{1:200}$$

$$= \frac{2.5 \text{ mg}}{1:200}$$

$$= \frac{2.5 \text{ mg}}{(1 \text{ g}/200 \text{ mL})}$$

$$= \frac{2.5 \text{ mg}}{(1{,}000 \text{ mg}/200 \text{ mL})}$$

$$= \frac{2.5 \text{ mg}}{5 \text{ mg}/\text{mL}}$$

$$= 0.5 \text{ mL}$$

EXERCISE 1   How many mg of active ingredient are in 0.5 mL of a 0.5% albuterol sulfate solution?

[Answer: Dosage = 2.5 mg]

EXERCISE 2   What volume is needed from a 0.5% solution in order to obtain 5 mg of active ingredient?

[Answer: Volume = 1 mL]

REFERENCE   Gardenhire

SEE   *Dosage Calculation: Unit Dose.*

SELF-ASSESSMENT QUESTIONS

23a. A 1:1,000 (0.1%) drug solution is the same as:

(A) 0.01 mg/mL.
(B) 0.1 mg/mL.
(C) 1 mg/mL.
(D) 10 mg/mL.

23b. How many mg of active ingredient are present in 0.5 mL of a 1:100 (1%) drug solution?

(A) 5 mg
(B) 10 mg
(C) 15 mg
(D) 20 mg

23c. How many mg of active ingredient are in 1 mL of a 1:200 drug solution?

(A) 1 mg
(B) 2 mg
(C) 5 mg
(D) 10 mg

23d. A 30-mL stock bottle of racemic epinephrine has a concentration of 2.25%. How much volume should be drawn from the bottle if 10 mg of the active ingredient are needed?

(A) 0.12 mL
(B) 0.25 mL
(C) 0.36 mL
(D) 0.44 mL

23e. How many mg of active ingredient are present in 0.25 mL of a 2.25% racemic epinephrine solution?

(A) 5.6 mg
(B) 6.4 mg
(C) 7.2 mg
(D) 8.8 mg

23f. What volume is needed from a 0.5% drug solution in order to obtain 5 mg of active ingredient?

(A) 0.25 mL
(B) 0.5 mL
(C) 1 mL
(D) 1.5 mL

23g. A stock bottle of acetylcysteine (Mucomyst) has a concentration of 10%. How many mg of active ingredient are present if 2 mL of this drug are used?

(A) 5 mg
(B) 10 mg
(C) 20 mg
(D) 200 mg

23h. How much of a 20% solution of acetylcysteine (Mucomyst) is needed in order to obtain 200 mg of active ingredient?

(A) 0.25 mL
(B) 0.5 mL
(C) 1 mL
(D) 1.5 mL

23i. The physician orders 0.15 mL of racemic epinephrine with normal saline for a child admitted for croup. If the racemic epinephrine solution has a concentration of 2.25%, about how much active ingredient is ordered?

(A) 0.34 mg
(B) 1.57 mg
(C) 2.25 mg
(D) 3.38 mg

Chapter

24

Dosage Calculation: Unit Dose

EQUATION 1   Dosage = Volume used × Concentration of unit dose

EQUATION 2 $\text{Volume} = \dfrac{\text{Dosage desired}}{\text{Concentration of unit dose}}$

EXAMPLE 1   A 2.5 mL unit dose of drug has a concentration of 0.2%. How many mg of active ingredient are in this unit dose? SOLUTION A. (This calculation gives an answer in g. It must be converted to mg.)

Dosage = Volume used × Concentration of unit dose
        = 2.5 mL × 0.2%
        = 2.5 mL × 0.002 g/mL
        = 0.005 g (or 5 mg)

SOLUTION B. The 0.2% solution can be rewritten as follows:

$0.2\% = \dfrac{0.2 \text{ g}}{100 \text{ mL}}$

$= \dfrac{200 \text{ mg}}{100 \text{ mg}}$

$= 2 \text{ mg/mL}$

(This calculation gives an answer in mg.)

Dosage = Volume used × Concentration of unit dose
        = 2.5 mL × 0.2%
        = 2.5 mL × 2 mg/mL
        = 5 mg

EXAMPLE 2   A unit dose of albuterol sulfate contains 3.0 mL in a 0.83 mg/mL concentration. How many mg of active ingredient are in this unit dose?

Dosage = Volume used × Concentration of unit dose
        = 3.0 mL × 0.83 mg/mL
        = 2.49 or 2.5 mg

EXAMPLE 3

A unit dose of albuterol sulfate contains 3.0 mL in a 0.83 mg/mL concentration. How much volume is needed if 1.5 mg of the active ingredient is desired?

$$\text{Volume} = \frac{\text{Dosage desired}}{\text{Concentration of unit dose}}$$

$$= \frac{1.5 \text{ mg}}{0.83 \text{ mg/mL}}$$

$$= 1.8 \text{ mL}$$

EXERCISE 1

A unit dose contains 2.5 mL in a 0.6% concentration. How many mg of active ingredient are in this unit dose? How much active ingredient is in half a unit dose?

[Answer: Dosage = 15 mg; $\frac{1}{2}$ unit dose = 7.5 mg]

EXERCISE 2

A unit dose of albuterol sulfate has 3.0 mL in a concentration of 0.042%. What is the total amount of active ingredient in this unit dose?

[Answer: Dosage in 3.0 mL = 1.26 mg]

EXERCISE 3

A 3.0 mL unit dose of albuterol sulfate has a concentration of 0.83 mg/mL. How much of this unit dose should be used if 1.66 mg of active ingredient are needed?

[Answer: Volume of unit dose needed = 2 mL]

REFERENCE

Gardenhire

SELF-ASSESSMENT QUESTIONS

24a. A unit dose of bronchodilator contains 5.0 mL in a 0.5 mg/mL concentration. How much active ingredient is in this unit dose?

(A) 0.5 mg
(B) 1.0 mg
(C) 2.5 mg
(D) 5.0 mg

24b. A unit dose of drug contains 2.5 mL in a 0.2% concentration. How many mg of active ingredient are present in this unit dose?

(A) 1.25 mg
(B) 2.5 mg
(C) 5 mg
(D) 10 mg

24c. A unit dose of Xopenex contains 3.0 mL in a 0.0417% concentration. How many mg of active ingredient are present in this unit dose?

(A) 0.75 mg

(B) 1.25 mg

(C) 0.63 mg

(D) 0.31 mg

24d. A unit dose of levalbuterol HCl contains 3.0 mL in a 0.0417% concentration. How many unit doses are needed in order to obtain 10 mg of the active ingredient?

(A) 4 unit doses

(B) 6 unit doses

(C) 8 unit doses

(D) 10 unit doses

24e. A unit dose contains 2.5 mL in a 0.6% concentration. How many mg of active ingredient are in this unit dose?

(A) 2.5 mg

(B) 5 mg

(C) 10 mg

(D) 15 mg

24f. A unit dose of albuterol sulfate contains 3.0 mL in a 0.083% concentration. If eight unit doses are used in a large-volume aerosol treatment, what is the total amount of active ingredient in the nebulizer?

(A) 2.5 mg

(B) 5 mg

(C) 10 mg

(D) 20 mg

24g. A 3-mL unit dose of levalbuterol HCl contains 0.63 mg of active ingredient. If 2 unit doses are used, how many mg of active ingredient are used?

(A) 1.26 mg

(B) 2.40 mg

(C) 2.86 mg

(D) 3.14 mg

24h. Each ampule of Brethine (terbutaline sulfate) contains 1 mL of a 0.1% solution. What is the total dosage if two ampules (2 mL) are used?

(A) 1 mg

(B) 2 mg

(C) 3 mg

(D) 4 mg

24i. The physician orders 0.5 mL of a unit dose of Brethine (terbutaline sulfate) with saline for a pediatric patient. If the 1 mL unit dose ampule comes in a 0.1% solution, how many mg of this drug are used?

(A) 0.01 mg

(B) 0.1 mg

(C) 0.5 mg

(D) 1.0 mg

24j. An ipratropium bromide unit dose contains 2.5 mL in a 0.02% concentration. How many mg of active ingredient are in a unit dose?

(A) 0.5 mg

(B) 1.0 mg

(C) 1.5 mg

(D) 5 mg

24k. The physician orders two unit doses of metaproterenol sulfate. If each unit dose contains 2.5 mL in a 0.4% concentration, how many mg of metaproterenol sulfate are ordered?

(A) 1 mg

(B) 2 mg

(C) 5 mg

(D) 10 mg

24l. A unit dose of liquid Intal (cromolyn sodium) contains 20 mg/2 mL. How much active ingredient is in 1 mL of this solution?

(A) 10 mg

(B) 15 mg

(C) 20 mg

(D) 40 mg

24m. What is the concentration in % if each 2-mL unit dose of cromolyn sodium contains 20 mg of active ingredient?

(A) 0.1%

(B) 1%

(C) 10%

(D) 5%

25

Dosage Estimation for Children: Young's Rule

NOTES

Young's rule of dosage calculation requires the child's *age*. It should be used for children ranging from 1 to 12 years of age.

If the child's weight is not in proportion to age, Clark's rule for dosage calculation should be used. See Dosage Estimation for Infants and Children: Clark's Rule.

Since an effective drug dosage varies greatly among individuals and conditions, the calculated dosage must be carefully evaluated before drug administration.

EQUATION

$$\text{Child's dose} = \left[\frac{\text{Age}}{(\text{Age} + 12)}\right] \times \text{Adult dose}$$

Child's dose : Estimated child's drug dosage

Age : Age of child in years

Adult dose : Normal adult drug dosage

EXAMPLE

What should be the dosage for an 8-year-old if the adult dose is 50 mg?

$$\text{Child's dose} = \left[\frac{\text{Age}}{(\text{Age} + 12)}\right] \times \text{Adult dose}$$

$$= \left[\frac{8}{(8 + 12)}\right] \times 50 \text{ mg}$$

$$= \left[\frac{8}{20}\right] \times 50 \text{ mg}$$

$$= 0.4 \times 50 \text{ mg}$$

$$= 20 \text{ mg}$$

EXERCISE

If the adult dose is 30 mg, what is the calculated pediatric dose for a 6-year-old patient?

[Answer: Dosage = 10 mg]

REFERENCE

Hegstad

SELF-ASSESSMENT QUESTIONS

25a. If the child's age is known and is within the range of 1 to 12 years, the drug dosage for this child can be estimated by using:

(A) Old's rule.

(B) Young's rule.

(C) Clark's rule.

(D) Fried's rule.

25b. If the drug dosage for an adult is 15 mg, what is the pediatric dosage for a 6-year-old patient using Young's rule for dosage calculation?

(A) 1 mg
(B) 2 mg
(C) 5 mg
(D) 10 mg

25c. Using Young's rule of dosage calculation for children, what should be the dosage for a 5-year-old child if the adult dose of a medication is 10 mg?

(A) 1.88 or 1.9 mg
(B) 2.45 or 2.5 mg
(C) 2.94 or 2.9 mg
(D) 3.07 or 3.1 mg

25d. If the adult dosage of a medication is 25 mg, what should be the dosage for a 10-year-old child based on Young's rule?

(A) 11.36 or 11 mg
(B) 12.41 or 12 mg
(C) 13.09 or 13 mg
(D) 14.44 or 14 mg

Chapter

26

Dosage Estimation for Infants and Children: Clark's Rule

NOTES

Clark's rule of dosage calculation requires the infant's or child's *weight*. Clark's rule can be used in infants and children. It provides a more reasonable estimate of drug dosage than Young's rule when the patient's body weight is not in proportion to age.

Because an effective drug dosage varies greatly among individuals and conditions, the calculated dosage must be carefully evaluated before drug administration.

EQUATION

$$\text{Infant's or child's dose} = \left[\frac{\text{Weight in lb}}{150}\right] \times \text{Adult dose}$$

Infant's or child's dose	: Estimated infant's or child's dosage
Weight in lb	: Weight of infant or child in pounds
Adult dose	: Normal adult drug dosage
150	: A constant number

EXAMPLE

What should be the dosage for a 50-lb child if the adult dose is 30 mg?

$$\text{Infant's or child's dose} = \left[\frac{\text{Weight in lb}}{150}\right] \times \text{Adult dose}$$

$$= \left[\frac{50}{150}\right] \times 30 \text{ mg}$$

$$= \frac{1}{3} \times 30 \text{ mg}$$

$$= 10 \text{ mg}$$

EXERCISE

If the adult dose is 50 mg, what is the calculated dosage for a 3-lb infant?

[Answer: Dosage = 1 mg]

REFERENCE

Hegstad

SELF-ASSESSMENT QUESTIONS

26a. With Clark's rule of dosage calculation for infants and children, what should be the dosage for a 6-lb infant if the adult dose is 30 mg?

(A) 1.2 mg

(B) 1.8 mg

(C) 2.4 mg

(D) 3.0 mg

26b. Use Clark's rule of dosage calculation for infants and children to calculate the dosage for a 50-lb child. The normal adult dose is 30 mg.

(A) 2 mg

(B) 5 mg

(C) 10 mg

(D) 20 mg

26c. If the weight of an infant or child is known, the drug dosage for this infant or child can be estimated by using:

(A) Young's rule.

(B) Rules of sevens.

(C) Clark's rule.

(D) Pickwick's rule.

27

Dosage Estimation for Infants and Children: Fried's Rule

NOTES

Fried's rule of dosage calculation requires the infant's or child's *age in months*. Fried's rule can be used for infants and children up to two years of age.

If the body weight of the infant or child is not in proportion to age, Clark's rule for dosage calculation should be used.

Since an effective drug dosage varies greatly among individuals and conditions, the calculated dosage must be carefully evaluated before drug administration.

EQUATION

$$\text{Infant's or child's dose} = \left(\frac{\text{Age in months}}{150} \right) \times \text{Adult dose}$$

Infant's or child's dose	:	Estimated infant's or child's dosage
Age in months	:	Age of infant or child in months, up to 24 months
Adult dose	:	Normal adult drug dosage
150	:	A constant number

EXAMPLE

What should be the dosage for a 15-month-old child if the adult dose is 30 mg?

$$\text{Infant's or child's dose} = \left(\frac{\text{Age in months}}{150} \right) \times \text{Adult dose}$$

$$= \left(\frac{15}{150} \right) \times 30 \text{ mg}$$

$$= \frac{1}{10} \times 30 \text{ mg}$$

$$= 3 \text{ mg}$$

EXERCISE

If the adult dose is 50 mg, what is the calculated dosage for a 2-year-old child?

[Answer: Dosage = 8 mg]

REFERENCE

Hegstad

SEE

Dosage Estimation for Infants and Children: Clark's Rule.

SELF-ASSESSMENT QUESTIONS

27a. Based on Fried's rule, what should be the dosage for a 2-year-old toddler if the adult dose is 35 mg?

(A) 3.9 mg

(B) 4.7 mg

(C) 5.1 mg

(D) 5.6 mg

27b. Use Fried's rule to estimate the dosage for a 15-month-old infant if the adult dose is 30 mg.

(A) 1 mg

(B) 2 mg

(C) 3 mg

(D) 4 mg

27c. According to Fried's rule, the estimated dosage for a 5-month-old infant based on an adult dose of 30 mg is:

(A) 1 mg.

(B) 2 mg.

(C) 3 mg.

(D) 4 mg.

27d. For infants and children up to two years old, the age in months may be used to estimate the drug dosage by using:

(A) Young's rule.

(B) Starling's rule.

(C) Clark's rule.

(D) Fried's rule.

Chapter

28

Elastance (E)

NOTES

The elastance equation is modified from Hooke's law of elastic behavior, and it is expressed as the reciprocal of compliance.

When the lungs are stiff (non-compliant), the elastance (E) of the lungs is high, and a high inflating pressure (ΔP) is required to deliver a set volume (ΔV). On the other hand, when the lungs are compliant, as in emphysema, the elastance of the lungs is low. In this situation, a high inflating pressure may be detrimental to the patient (e.g., barotrauma).

Compliance (C) is more commonly used to describe the elastic properties of the lungs.

EQUATION

$$E = \frac{\Delta P}{\Delta V}$$

E : Elastance in cm H_2O/L
ΔP : Pressure change in cm H_2O
ΔV : Volume change in mL or L

NORMAL VALUE

5 to 10 cm H_2O/L

If the patient is intubated, use serial measurements to establish trend.

EXAMPLE

Given: ΔP = 5 cm H_2O
    ΔV = 0.8 L
Calculate the elastance.

$$E = \frac{\Delta P}{\Delta V}$$
$$= \frac{5}{0.8}$$
$$= 6.25 \text{ cm } H_2O/L$$

EXERCISE

Given: ΔP = 3 cm H_2O
    ΔV = 0.6 L
Calculate the elastance.

[Answer: E = 5 cm H_2O/L]

REFERENCE

Wilkins (2)

SEE

Compliance: Dynamic (C_{dyn}); Compliance: Static (C_{st}).

SELF-ASSESSMENT QUESTIONS

28a. Calculate the elastance if the change in pressure (ΔP) is 10 cm H_2O and change in volume (ΔV) is 0.5 L. Is it normal?

    (A) 20 cm H_2O/L; abnormal

    (B) 10 cm H_2O/L; normal

    (C) 5 cm H_2O/L; normal

    (D) 10 L/cm H_2O; abnormal

$$\frac{10}{0.5} = 20$$

28b. Calculate the elastance if the change in pressure (ΔP) is 5 cm H_2O and change in volume (ΔV) is 0.7 L. Is it normal?

    (A) 3.5 cm H_2O/L; abnormal

    (B) 5 cm H_2O/L; normal

    (C) 7.1 cm H_2O/L; normal

    (D) 8.9 L/cm H_2O; abnormal

$$\frac{5}{0.7} =$$

28c. Which of the following patient conditions has the lowest elastance?

    (A) Atelectasis

    (B) Emphysema

    (C) Pulmonary fibrosis

    (D) Consolidation

28d. Elastance is the opposite of:

    (A) reliance.

    (B) resistance.

    (C) conductance.

    (D) compliance.

Chapter

29

Endotracheal Tube Size for Children

NOTES

This equation is used to estimate the size of an endotracheal (ET) tube for a child more than one year of age. The calculated size should be adjusted up or down by 0.5 mm for different body sizes. In an emergency situation, an ET tube may be selected by matching one with the diameter of a child's little finger.

Because ET tubes come in 0.5-mm increments, the estimated *ID* size should be rounded to the nearest whole or half size.

For neonates, the endotracheal tube size is not calculated. Rather, Table 2-4 shows the general rule for selecting an appropriate endotracheal tube for a neonate.

EQUATION 1

$$ID = \frac{Age + 16}{4}$$

or

EQUATION 2

$$ID = \frac{Height}{20}$$

ID : Internal diameter of endotracheal tube in mm
Age : Age of child over one year of age, in years
Height : Height of child in cm

EXAMPLE 1

What is the estimated size of an endotracheal tube for a 3-year-old child?

$$ID = \frac{Age + 16}{4}$$
$$= \frac{3 + 16}{4}$$
$$= \frac{19}{4}$$
$$= 4.75 \text{ or } 5.0 \text{ mm}$$

EXAMPLE 2

What is the estimated size of an endotracheal tube for a child who is 4 ft* (about 120 cm) tall?

$$ID = \frac{Height}{20}$$
$$= \frac{120}{20}$$
$$1 = 6.0 \text{ mm}$$

EXERCISE 1

Calculate the estimated ET tube size for a 6-year-old child.

[Answer: *ID* = 5.5 mm]

*1 *ft* = 12 *in.* and 1 *in.* = 2.54 *cm.*

TABLE 2-4. Endotracheal Tube Size for Neonates

BODY WEIGHT	ET SIZE (*ID mm*)
<1,000 g	2.5
1,000 to 2,000 g	3.0
2,000 to 3,000 g	3.5
>3,000 g	4.0

EXERCISE 2   Calculate the estimated ET tube size for a child 3 ft (90 cm) tall.

[Answer: *ID* = 4.5 mm]

REFERENCES   Koff; Whitaker

SELF-ASSESSMENT QUESTIONS

29a. Calculate the estimated size of an endotracheal tube for a 2-year-old child.

 (A) 4 mm
 (B) 4.5 mm
 (C) 5 mm
 (D) 5.5 mm

$$\frac{2 + 16}{4} = \frac{18}{4} = 4.5 \text{ mm}$$

29b. For an 8-year-old child, the calculated size of an endotracheal tube is about:

 (A) 5 mm.
 (B) 5.5 mm.
 (C) 6 mm.
 (D) 6.5 mm.

$$\frac{8 + 16}{4} = \frac{24}{4} = 6 \text{ mm}$$

29c. Calculate the estimated size of an endotracheal tube for a child who is 3'6" (about 106 cm) tall.

 (A) 3.5 mm
 (B) 4 mm
 (C) 4.5 mm
 (D) 5 mm

$$\frac{106}{20} = 5 \text{ mm}$$

29d. What should be the size of an endotracheal tube for a child who is 2'6" (about 76 cm) tall?

 (A) 3.5 mm
 (B) 4 mm
 (C) 4.5 mm
 (D) 5 mm

30

Fick's Law of Diffusion

NOTES

Gas diffusion rate is directly related to the cross-sectional area of the lung membrane, the diffusion coefficient of gas, and the pressure gradient. It is inversely related to the thickness across the lung membrane.

EQUATION

$$\text{Diffusion} = \frac{A \times D \times \Delta P}{T}$$

Diffusion : Gas diffusion rate

A : Cross-sectional area of lung membrane
In emphysema, some lung tissues are destroyed, and the overall cross-sectional area of the lungs is diminished. The diffusion rate for these patients measured in the pulmonary function laboratory is therefore usually low.

D : Diffusion coefficient of a gas
Carbon monoxide (CO) is used in gas diffusion studies because of its high diffusion rate and its ability to combine readily with hemoglobin (250 times greater than that of oxygen). CO is known as a diffusion-limited gas because its diffusion rate in the lungs is limited only by conditions in which the cross-sectional area of the lung membrane or the thickness across the lung membrane is affected.

ΔP : Pressure gradient of a gas
Pressure gradient of a gas is the fundamental principle of gas diffusion and exchange. Gas diffusion in the lungs and in the tissues follows the basic rule of pressure gradient: from an area of high pressure to an area of low pressure. In the pulmonary circulation, oxygen diffuses from alveoli ($P_A O_2 >$ 100 mm Hg) to pulmonary capillaries $\left(P_{\bar{v}} O_2 = 40 \text{ mm Hg}\right)$, and carbon dioxide diffuses from pulmonary capillaries $\left(P_{\bar{v}} CO_2 = 46 \text{ mm Hg}\right)$ to alveoli ($P_A CO_2 = 40$ mm Hg). Oxygen therapy relies on this principle by increasing the pressure gradient of oxygen between the alveoli and pulmonary capillaries. A higher oxygen diffusion gradient facilitates oxygen diffusion into the pulmonary capillaries, and oxygenation of the mixed venous blood is therefore enhanced.

T : Thickness across lung membrane
Gas diffusion is hindered when the thickness across the lung membrane is increased. Pulmonary or interstitial edema, consolidation, and pulmonary fibrosis are some clinical conditions accompanied by an increase in thickness across the lung membrane. Oxygen therapy is not very effective in these conditions because oxygen, having a low diffusion coefficient, cannot diffuse across these lung units very well.

REFERENCES   Des Jardins; Wilkins (2)

SEE   *Graham's Law of Diffusion Coefficient.*

SELF-ASSESSMENT QUESTIONS

30a. The diffusion rate of oxygen across the alveolar-capillary membrane is directly related to all of the following factors *except*:

(A) diffusion coefficient of oxygen.
(B) cross-sectional area of lung membrane.
(C) alveolar-capillary pressure gradient of oxygen.
(D) thickness across lung membrane.

30b. In emphysema patients, the diffusion rate of gases across the alveolar-capillary membrane is lower than normal primarily because of:

(A) airway obstruction.
(B) hypoventilation.
(C) acidosis.
(D) reduction of cross-sectional area of lung membrane.

30c. In a pulmonary function laboratory, the gas diffusion rate is usually determined by using _____ because of its _____ diffusion coefficient.

(A) carbon monoxide; high
(B) carbon monoxide; low
(C) oxygen; high
(D) oxygen; low

30d. Under normal conditions, the pressure gradient of oxygen between the arterial and mixed venous blood is about _____ mm Hg, considerably _____ than the pressure gradient of carbon dioxide.

(A) 60; lower
(B) 60; higher
(C) 40; lower
(D) 40; higher

30e. A patient who is diagnosed with pneumonia has retained a large amount of secretions. This condition hinders gas diffusion and causes hypoxemia as a result of an increase of the:

(A) diffusion coefficient of oxygen.
(B) cross-sectional area of lung membrane.
(C) pressure gradient of oxygen.
(D) thickness across lung membrane.

Chapter

31

F_IO_2 from Two Gas Sources

NOTE

This equation is useful when a special oxygen setup involves two gas sources, and an oxygen analyzer is not readily available.

EQUATION

$$F_IO_2 = \frac{(1st\ F_IO_2 \times 1st\ flow) + (2nd\ F_IO_2 \times 2nd\ flow)}{Total\ flow}$$

F_IO_2 : Inspired oxygen concentration in %

1st F_IO_2 : Oxygen concentration of 1st gas source in %

1st flow : Flow rate of 1st gas source in L/min

2nd F_IO_2 : Oxygen concentration of 2nd gas source in %

2nd flow : Flow rate of 2nd gas source in L/min

EXAMPLE 1

What is the final F_IO_2 if 8 L/min of air is mixed with 2 L/min of oxygen?

$$
\begin{aligned}
F_IO_2 &= \frac{(1st\ F_IO_2 \times 1st\ flow) + (2nd\ F_IO_2 \times 2nd\ flow)}{Total\ flow} \\
&= \frac{(0.21 \times 8) + (1.00 \times 2)}{(8 + 2)} \\
&= \frac{1.68 + 2}{10} \\
&= \frac{3.68}{10} \\
&= 0.368\ or\ 37\%
\end{aligned}
$$

EXAMPLE 2

If the oxygen:air entrainment ratio is 1:10, what is the F_IO_2?

$$
\begin{aligned}
F_IO_2 &= \frac{(1st\ F_IO_2 \times 1st\ flow) + (2nd\ F_IO_2 \times 2nd\ flow)}{Total\ flow} \\
&= \frac{(1.00 \times 1) + (0.21 \times 10)}{(1 + 10)} \\
&= \frac{1 + 2.1}{11} \\
&= \frac{3.1}{11} \\
&= 0.28\ or\ 28\%
\end{aligned}
$$

EXAMPLE 3   Calculate the F_IO_2 when 6 L/min of 40% oxygen is mixed with 2 L/min of air.

$$F_IO_2 = \frac{\left(\text{1st } F_IO_2 \times \text{1st flow}\right) + \left(\text{2nd } F_IO_2 \times \text{2nd flow}\right)}{\text{Total flow}}$$

$$= \frac{(0.40 \times 6) + (0.21 \times 2)}{(6 + 2)}$$

$$= \frac{2.4 + 0.42}{8}$$

$$= \frac{2.82}{8}$$

$$= 0.353 \text{ or } 35\%$$

EXERCISE 1   If 3 L/min of 28% oxygen is mixed with 6 L/min of air, what is the final F_IO_2?

[Answer: F_IO_2 = 0.233 or 23%]

EXERCISE 2   Calculate the F_IO_2 when 6 L/min of 60% oxygen is mixed with 4 L/min of air.

[Answer: F_IO_2 = 0.444 or 44%]

REFERENCE   Barnes

SEE   *Oxygen:Air (O_2:Air) Entrainment Ratio.*

SELF-ASSESSMENT QUESTIONS

31a. What is the oxygen concentration if 5 L/min of air is mixed with 5 L/min of oxygen?

(A) 30%
(B) 40%
(C) 50%
(D) 60%

31b. What is the approximate F_IO_2 when 6 L/min of air is mixed with 2 L/min of oxygen?

(A) 30%
(B) 35%
(C) 40%
(D) 45%

31c. Calculate the F_IO_2 when 1 L/min of oxygen is mixed with 4 L/min of air.

(A) 32%
(B) 37%
(C) 41%
(D) 46%

31d. If the oxygen:air entrainment ratio is 1:10, what is F_IO_2?

(A) 22%

(B) 24%

(C) 26%

(D) 28%

31e. Which of the following oxygen:air entrainment ratios provides an F_IO_2 of 60%?

(A) 1:0.5

(B) 1:1

(C) 1:1.5

(D) 1:2

Chapter

32

F_IO_2 Needed for a Desired P_aO_2

NOTES

This two-step calculation is used to estimate the F_IO_2 needed to obtain a desired P_aO_2.

This calculation is useful to estimate the F_IO_2 needed in hypoxemia caused by hypoventilation or venous admixture (V/Q mismatch). In severe intrapulmonary shunts, this method is less dependable; positive end-expiratory pressure (PEEP) or continuous positive airway pressure (CPAP) may be needed for corrections of intrapulmonary shunting.

For unusual P_aCO_2 or barometric pressure (P_B), use the F_IO_2 equation that follows.

$$F_IO_2 = \frac{P_AO_2 \text{ needed} + \left(P_aCO_2 \times 1.25\right)}{P_B - 47}$$

EQUATION 1

$$P_AO_2 \text{ needed} = \frac{P_aO_2 \text{ desired}}{a/A \text{ ratio*}}$$

EQUATION 2

$$F_IO_2 = \frac{P_AO_2 \text{ needed} + 50}{713}$$

P_AO_2 needed : Alveolar oxygen tension needed for a desired P_aO_2

P_aO_2 desired : Arterial oxygen tension desired

a/A ratio : Arterial/alveolar oxygen tension ratio in %

F_IO_2 : Inspired oxygen concentration needed to get a desired P_aO_2

EXAMPLE

Given: a/A ratio = 0.55. What should be the F_IO_2 if a P_aO_2 of 100 mm Hg is desired?

(1) P_AO_2 needed $= \dfrac{P_aO_2 \text{ desired}}{a/A \text{ ratio*}}$

$= \dfrac{100}{0.55}$

$= 182$ mm hg

(2) F_IO_2 needed $= \dfrac{P_AO_2 \text{ needed} + 50}{713}$

$= \dfrac{182 + 50}{713}$

$= \dfrac{232}{713}$

$= 0.325$ or 33%

EXERCISE

Given: a/A ratio = 0.30. What should be the F_IO_2 if a P_aO_2 of 80 mm Hg is desired?

[Answer: F_IO_2 = 0.44 or 44%]

REFERENCES

Wilkins (2)

Arterial/Alveolar Oxygen Tension (a/A) Ratio.

SELF-ASSESSMENT QUESTIONS

32a. Given: a/A ratio = 0.35. What should be the F_IO_2 if a P_aO_2 of 100 mm Hg is desired?

(A) 27%

(B) 38%

(C) 47%

(D) 55%

32b. Given: a/A ratio = 0.35. What should be the F_IO_2 if a P_aO_2 of 50 mm Hg is desired?

(A) 27%

(B) 38%

(C) 47%

(D) 55%

32c. The a/A ratio in a patient is 0.80. If a P_aO_2 of 80 mm Hg is desired, what should be the F_IO_2? Is oxygen therapy necessary?

(A) 21%; not necessary

(B) 24%; necessary

(C) 28%; necessary

(D) 32%; necessary

Chapter

33

F_IO_2 Needed for a Desired P_aO_2 (COPD Patients)

NOTE

This calculation is used to estimate the F_IO_2 needed to obtain a low-range (50 to 60 mm Hg) P_aO_2, a value most suitable for COPD patients with uncomplicated acute exacerbation. To use this equation, a recent room air P_aO_2 must be known.

In this equation, the unit for P_aO_2 (mm Hg) is not used and is replaced by percent (%).

EQUATION

$$F_IO_2 = 21\% + \left[\frac{\left(P_aO_2 \text{ desired } - \text{ Room air } P_aO_2 \right)}{3} \right]\%$$

F_IO_2 : Inspired oxygen concentration needed to get a desired P_aO_2, in %

P_aO_2 desired : Arterial oxygen tension desired

Room air P_aO_2 : Arterial oxygen tension on 21% oxygen

EXAMPLE

Given: Room air P_aO_2 = 45 mm Hg. What should be the F_IO_2 if a P_aO_2 of 60 mm Hg is desired?

$$F_IO_2 = 21\% + \left[\frac{\left(P_aO_2 \text{ desired } - \text{ Room air } P_aO_2 \right)}{3} \right]\%$$

$$= 21\% + \left[\frac{(60 - 45)}{3} \right]\%$$

$$= 21\% + \left[\frac{15}{3} \right]\%$$

$$= 21\% + 5\%$$

$$= 26\%$$

EXERCISE

Given: Room air P_aO_2 = 35 mm Hg. Estimate the F_IO_2 needed for a P_aO_2 of 55 mm Hg.

[Answer: F_IO_2 = 28%]

REFERENCE

Malley

SELF-ASSESSMENT QUESTIONS

33a. The room air P_aO_2 of a COPD patient is 40 mm Hg. What should be the F_IO_2 if a P_aO_2 of 60 mm Hg is desired?

(A) 22%

(B) 24%

(C) 26%

(D) 28%

$$\frac{60 - 40}{3}$$

$21\% + 5 = 26\%$

$21\% + 6.6667 = 28\%$

33b. The P_aO_2 of a COPD patient is 40 mm Hg at an F_IO_2 of 21%. If
a P_aO_2 of 55 mm Hg is desired, calculate the F_IO_2 needed.

(A) 22%

(B) 24%

(C) 26%

(D) 28%

$$55 - 40 = 15 \div 3 = 5$$

$$21\% + 5\% = 26\%$$

33c. The typical baseline P_aO_2 for COPD should be maintained
between:

(A) 40 and 50 mm Hg.

(B) 50 and 60 mm Hg.

(C) 60 and 70 mm Hg.

(D) 70 and 80 mm Hg.

34

Flow Rate in Mechanical Ventilation

NOTES

This equation is used to calculate the *minimum* flow rate required in mechanical ventilation.

The calculated flow rate should be increased accordingly when the minute ventilation increases, as in IMV or Assist Mode. In addition, a longer expiratory time would require a higher flow rate.

Unless the patient's minute ventilation stays fairly consistent, the flow rate should be set 10 to 15 L/min higher than the calculated flow rate.

EQUATION

Minimum flow rate = $\dot{V}_E \times$ Sum of $I{:}E$ ratio

Minimum flow rate : Minimum flow rate required to provide certain minute ventilation and $I{:}E$ ratio, in L/min

$\dot{V}_E$: Expired minute ventilation in L/min ($V_T \times f$)

Sum of $I{:}E$ ratio   : The sum of the inspiratory:expiratory ratio

EXAMPLE

Given: V_T = 700 mL (0.7 L)
f = 16/min
$I{:}E$ ratio = 1:3

Calculate the minimum flow rate required for the above settings.

$$
\begin{aligned}
\text{Minimum flow rate} &= \dot{V}_E \times \text{Sum of } I{:}E \text{ ratio} \\
&= (V_T \times f) \times \text{Sum of } I{:}E \text{ ratio} \\
&= (0.7 \times 16) \times (1 + 3) \\
&= 11.2 \times 4 \\
&= 44.8 \text{ or } 45 \text{ L/min}
\end{aligned}
$$

EXERCISE

Given: V_T = 800 mL (0.8 L)
f = 12/min
$I{:}E$ ratio = 1:3

What is the minimum flow rate needed for the above settings?

[Answer: Minimum flow rate = 38 L/min]

REFERENCE

Dupuis

SEE

I:E Ratio.

SELF-ASSESSMENT QUESTIONS

34a. If the expired minute ventilation is 15 L/min and an $I:E$ ratio of 1:2.5 is desired, what should be the *minimum* flow rate required for the above settings?

(A) 42 L/min

(B) 46 L/min

(C) 50 L/min

(D) 53 L/min

34b. Given: V_T = 750 mL (0.75 L), f = 12/min, $I:E$ ratio = 1:3. What should be the *minimum* flow rate required for the above settings?

(A) 36 L/min

(B) 40 L/min

(C) 48 L/min

(D) 51 L/min

$$(0.75L \times 12) \times (1+3)$$
$$9 \times 4 = 36$$

34c. Given: V_T = 600 mL (0.6 L), f = 16/min, $I:E$ ratio = 1:3. What should be the *minimum* flow rate needed for these settings?

(A) 36 L/min

(B) 38 L/min

(C) 43 L/min

(D) 48 L/min

$$(0.6L \times 16) \times (1+3)$$
$$9.6 \times 4 = 38.4$$

Chapter

35

Forced Vital Capacity Tracing (FEV_t and $FEV_{t\%}$)

The method to find other FEV_t and $FEV_{t\%}$ measurements is the same as shown in Examples 1 and 2. For accurate results, it is extremely important to plot the points carefully and draw straight lines with a ruler.

The $FEV_{0.5}$ and $FEV_{1.0}$ (as well as $FEF_{200-1200}$) are used to assess the flow rates and disorders relating to the large airways. In patients with large airway obstruction, these values are decreased. However, poor patient effort may also lead to lower than normal results. The $FEV_{t\%}$ values are also reduced in patients with obstructive disorders.

In patients with restrictive lung disorders, essentially all FEV_t measurements are decreased. However, the $FEV_{t\%}$ may be normal or increased because of the concurrent decrease in FVC. For example, when $FEV_{1.0}$ and FVC are both decreased, the $FEV_{1.0\%}$ ($FEV_{1.0}$/FVC) may show little or no change.

EQUATION

FEV_t : Forced Expiratory Volume (timed), in liters (t is commonly expressed in 0.5, 1, 2, or 3 sec)

$FEV_{t\%}$: Forced Expiratory Volume (timed)/Forced Vital Capacity (FVC), in %

NORMAL VALUES

FEV_t

$FEV_{0.5}$ = 3.1 L
FEV_1 = 4.2 L
FEV_2 = 4.6 L
FEV_3 = 4.8 L

The FEV_t normal values are based on a 70", 20-year-old male. Since the normal predicted values are based on a person's gender, age, height, weight, smoking history, and ethnic origin, an appropriate normal table should be used to match a person's physical attributes.

$FEV_{t\%}$

$FEV_{0.5\%}$ = 50% to 60%
$FEV_{1\%}$ = 75% to 85%
$FEV_{2\%}$ = 94%
$FEV_{3\%}$ = 97%

$FEV_{t\%}$ expresses a person's FEV_t relative to the FVC. The $FEV_{t\%}$ normal values may be accepted for all subjects regardless of gender, age, height, and other physical attributes. For clinical evaluation of lung impairments, an $FEV_{1\%}$ of 65% or less is significant and diagnostic of airway obstruction.

EXAMPLE 1

From the PFT tracing (Figure 2-4), find $FEV_{0.5}$.
Step 1. Along the time (x) axis, locate 0.5 sec (point A).
Step 2. From point A, draw a vertical line upward until it intersects the PFT tracing (point B).
Step 3. From point B, draw a horizontal line until it intersects the volume (y) axis (point C).
Step 4. The reading at point C (0.85 L) is the volume expired during the first 0.5 sec of the FVC maneuver.
Therefore, $FEV_{0.5}$ = 0.85 L.

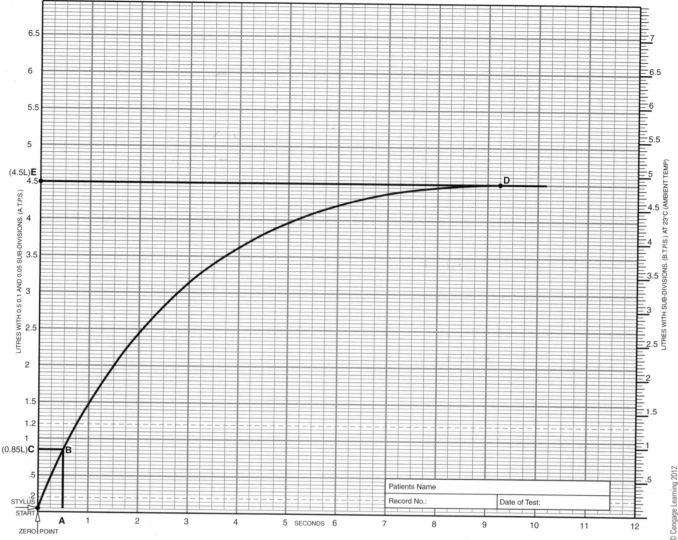

Figure 2-4 Examples to find FEV$_{0.5}$ and FEV$_{0.5\%}$.

EXAMPLE 2

From the PFT tracing (Figure 2-4), find FEV$_{0.5\%}$. Is the result normal?

Step 1. From the PFT tracing, locate the highest point at the end of the tracing (point D).

Step 2. From point D, draw a horizontal line until it intersects the volume (y) axis (point E).

Step 3. The reading at point E (4.5 L) represents the FVC.

$$FEV_{0.5\%} = FEV_{0.5}/FVC$$
$$= 0.85 \text{ L}/4.5 \text{ L}$$
$$= 0.1888$$
$$= 18.9\%$$

FEV$_{0.5\%}$ of 18.9% is below normal.

EXERCISE 1

From the PFT tracing (Figure 2-5), find FEV$_1$.

[Answer: FEV$_1$ = 2.4 L] (See Figure 2-6.)

EXERCISE 2   From the PFT tracing (Figure 2-5), find FEV$_{1\%}$. Is it normal?

[Answers: FEV$_{1\%}$ = 2.4/5.05 or 47.5%; the FEV$_{1\%}$ is lower than predicted] (See Figure 2-6.)

REFERENCE   Ruppel

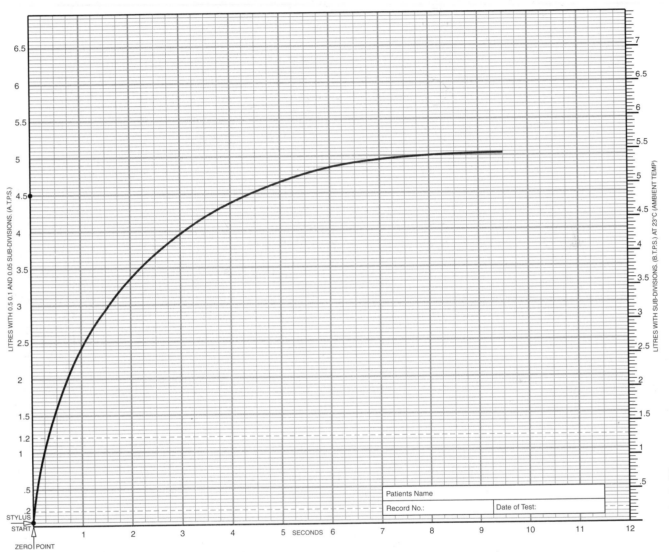

Figure 2-5 Exercises to find FEV$_1$ and FEV$_{1\%}$.

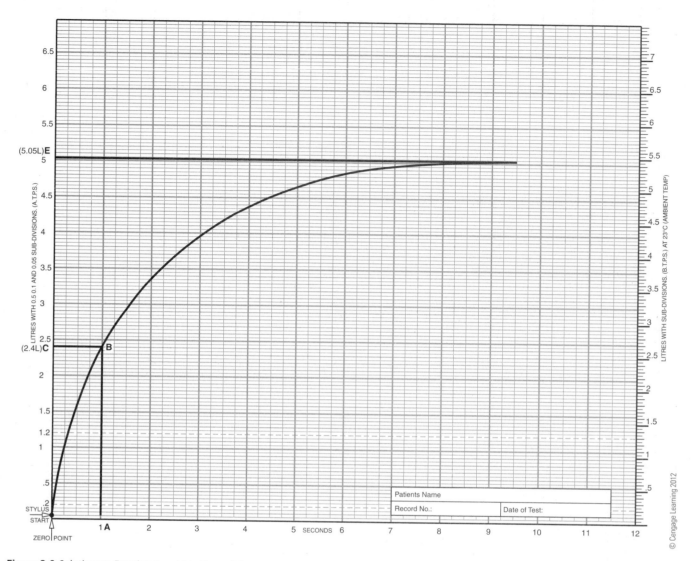

Figure 2-6 Solutions to Exercises 1 and 2 in Figure 2-5.

© Cengage Learning 2012

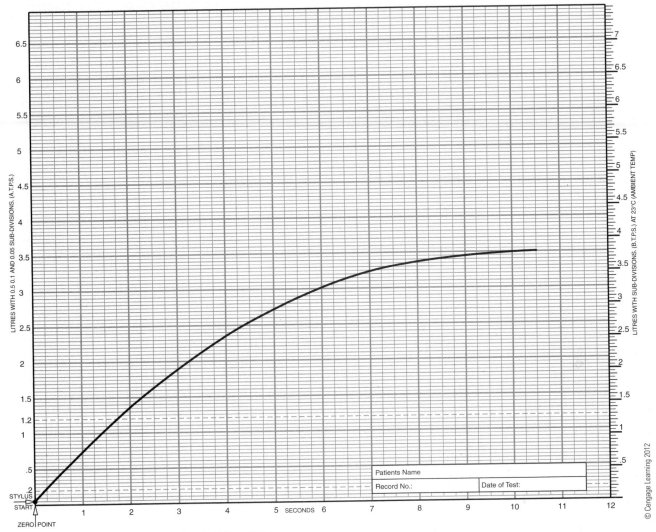

Figure 2-7 Self-assessment question to find FEV$_1$, FVC, and FEV$_{1\%}$.

SELF-ASSESSMENT QUESTIONS

35a. From the PFT tracing (Figure 2-7), find FEV$_1$, FVC, and FEV$_{1\%}$. Is the FEV$_{1\%}$ normal?

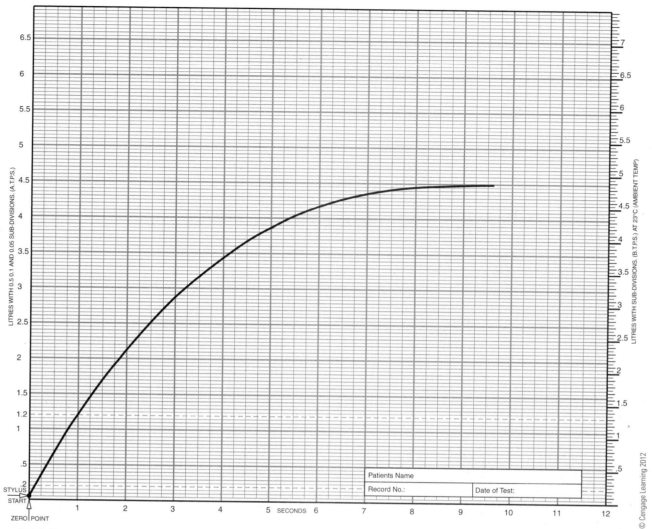

Figure 2-8 Self-assessment question to find FEV$_2$, FVC, and FEV$_{2\%}$.

35b. From the PFT tracing (Figure 2-8), find FEV$_2$, FVC, and FEV$_{2\%}$. Is the FEV$_{2\%}$ normal?

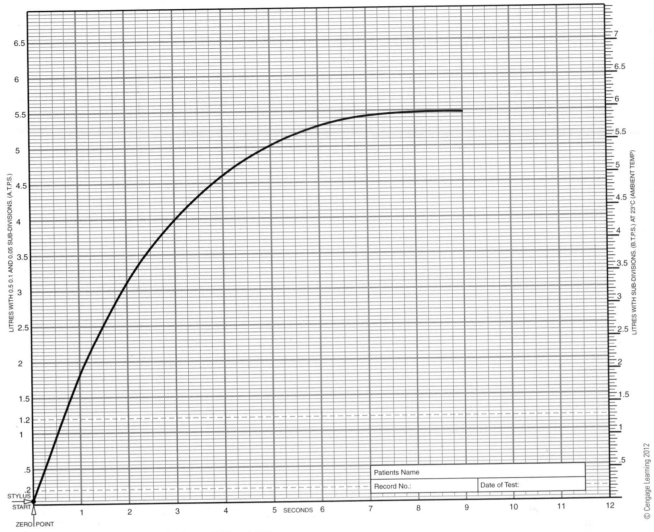

Figure 2-9 Self-assessment question to find FEV$_3$, FVC, and FEV$_{3\%}$.

35c. From the PFT tracing (Figure 2-9), find FEV$_3$, FVC, and FEV$_{3\%}$. Is the FEV$_{3\%}$ normal?

36

Forced Vital Capacity Tracing (FEF$_{200-1200}$)

NOTES

The FEF$_{200-1200}$ measurement is dependent on the slope derived from the PFT tracing. A steep PFT tracing results in a higher FEF$_{200-1200}$ measurement. The method to plot the slopes from other PFT tracings is the same as shown in Example 1. For accurate results, it is extremely important to plot the points precisely and draw straight lines with a ruler.

The FEF$_{200-1200}$ (as well as FEV$_{0.5}$ and FEV$_{1.0}$) is used to assess flow rates and disorders relating to the large airways. In patients with large airway obstruction, the FEF$_{200-1200}$ values are usually decreased. However, poor patient effort may also lead to lower-than-normal results.

EQUATION

FEF$_{200-1200}$:   Flow rate of the initial 200 to 1,200 mL of volume expired during the FVC maneuver, in L/sec.

NORMAL VALUE

FEF$_{200-1200}$ = 8.7 L/sec
This value is based on a 70", 20-year-old male. Since the normal predicted values are based on a person's gender, age, height, weight, smoking history, and ethnic origin, an appropriate normal table should be used to match a person's physical attributes.

EXAMPLE 1

From the PFT tracing (Figure 2-10), find FEF$_{200-1200}$.

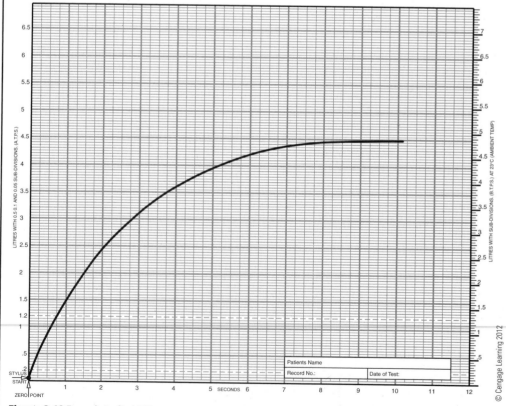

Figure 2-10 Example to find FEF$_{200-1200}$.

© Cengage Learning 2012

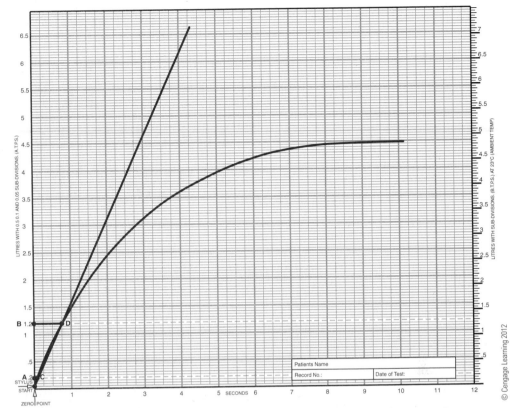

Figure 2-11 Locating the 0.2-L and 1.2-L markings on spirograph and determining its slope on graph paper.

Figure 2-11   Step 1. Along the volume (y) axis, locate 0.2 L (point A) and 1.2 L (point B).

Step 2. From point A, draw a horizontal line until it intersects the PFT tracing (point C). Do the same from point B until the line intersects the PFT tracing (point D).

Step 3. Use a ruler to draw a straight line connecting points C and D. Extend this straight line to top of the graph paper. This is the FEF$_{200-1200}$ flow slope.

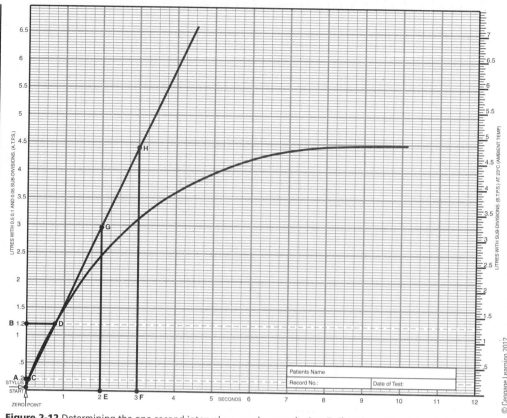

Figure 2-12 Determining the one-second interval on graph paper (points E, F) and spirograph tracing (points G, H).

Figure 2-12   Step 4. Along the time (x) axis, select two adjacent second-lines and mark them points E and F. In the example shown, the 2nd and 3rd second-lines are used. One may use the 3rd and 4th second-lines. The result would be identical as these two sets of adjacent lines intersect the same slope.

Step 5. From point E, follow the second line vertically until it intersects the slope (point G). Do the same from point F until it intersects the slope (point H).

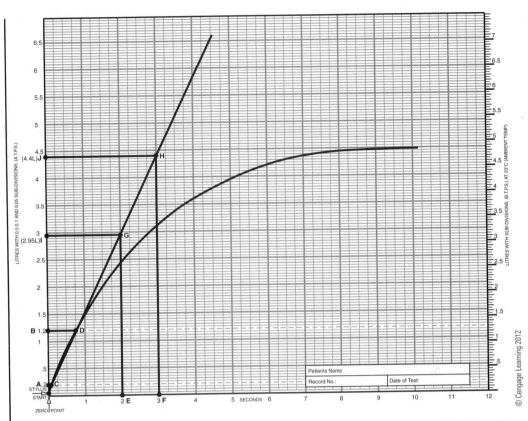

Figure 2-13 Determining the volume (L) that corresponds to the one-second interval (sec) on the slope. The unit of this reading is L/sec.

Figure 2-13   Step 6. From point G, draw a horizontal line until it intersects the volume (y) axis (point I). Do the same from point H until it intersects the volume (y) axis (point J).

Step 7. The difference between the volume readings taken at points I and J represents the flow rate of the initial 200 to 1200 mL of volume expired during the FVC maneuver.

$$FEF_{200-1200} = (4.4 \text{ L} - 2.95 \text{ L})/\text{sec}$$
$$= 1.45 \text{ L/sec}$$

EXERCISE   From the PFT tracing (Figure 2-14), find FEF$_{200-1200}$.

[Answer: FEF$_{200-1200}$ = (6.9 L − 3.5 L)/sec or 3.4 L/sec] (See Figure 2-15.)

REFERENCE   Ruppel

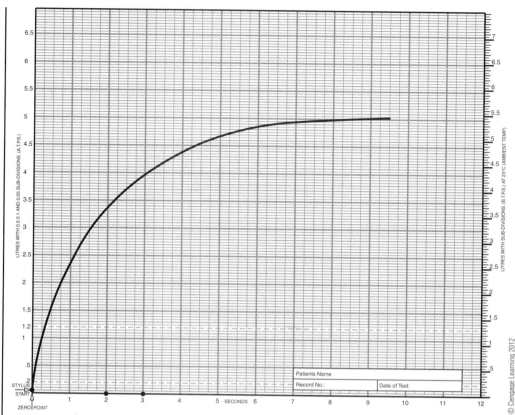

Figure 2-14 Exercise to find FEF$_{200-1200}$.

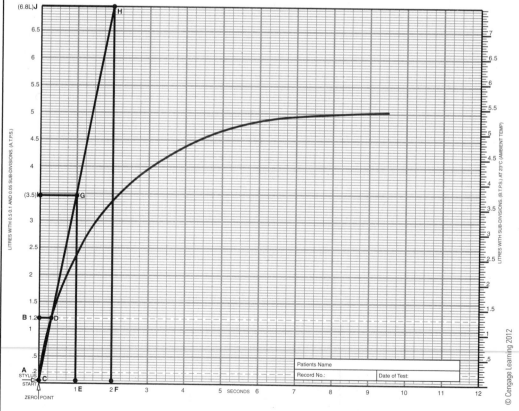

Figure 2-15 Solution to exercise in Figure 2-14.

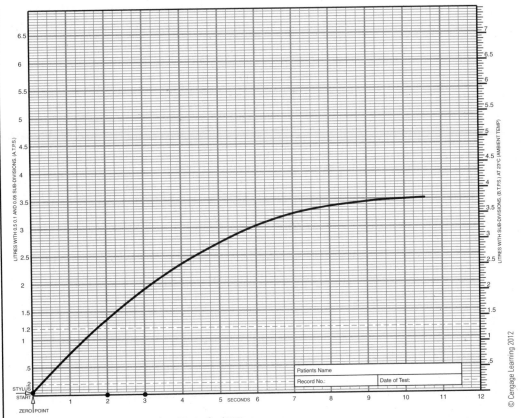

Figure 2-16 Self-assessment question 36a to find FEF$_{200-1200}$.

SELF-ASSESSMENT QUESTIONS

36a. From the PFT tracing (Figure 2-16), find FEF$_{200-1200}$.

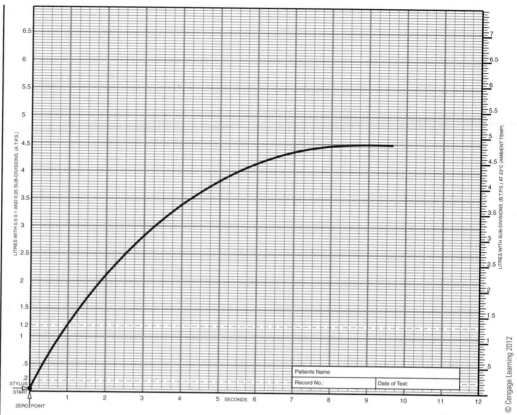

Figure 2-17 Self-assessment question 36b to find FEF$_{200-1200}$.

36b. From the PFT tracing (Figure 2-17), find FEF$_{200-1200}$.

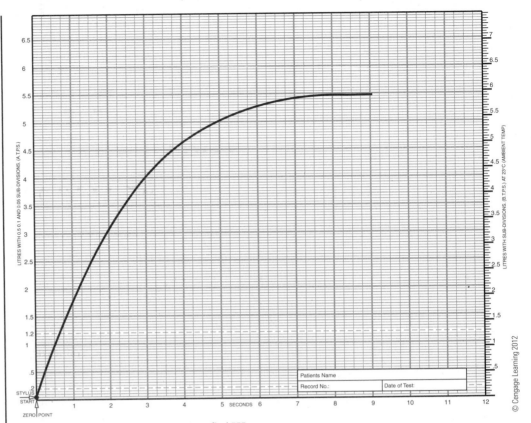

Figure 2-18 Self-assessment question 36c to find FEF$_{200-1200}$.

36c. From the PFT tracing (Figure 2-18), find FEF$_{200-1200}$.

37

Forced Vital Capacity Tracing (FEF$_{25-75\%}$)

NOTES

The method to plot the FEF$_{25-75\%}$ slopes from other PFT tracings is the same as shown in Example 1. For accurate results, it is extremely important to locate and plot the points carefully and draw straight lines using a ruler.

The FEF$_{25-75\%}$ (as well as FEV$_2$) is used to assess the flow rates and disorders relating to the smaller bronchi and larger bronchioles. In patients with early airway obstruction, the FEF$_{25-75\%}$ values are usually decreased. Patient effort has minimal effect on the FEF$_{25-75\%}$ measurements.

EQUATION

FEF$_{25-75\%}$: Flow rate of the middle 50% of the volume expired during the FVC maneuver, in L/sec.

NORMAL VALUES

FEF$_{25-75\%}$ = 5.2 L/sec
This value is based on a 70", 20-year-old male. As the normal predicted values are based on a person's gender, age, height, weight, smoking history, and ethnic origin, an appropriate normal table should be used to match a person's physical attributes.

EXAMPLE 1

From the PFT tracing (Figure 2-19), find FEF$_{25-75\%}$.

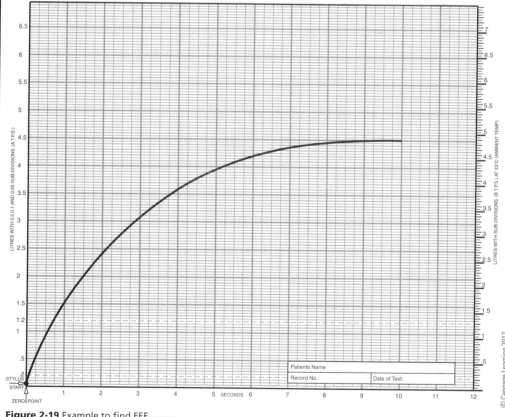

Figure 2-19 Example to find FEF$_{25-75\%}$.

© Cengage Learning 2012

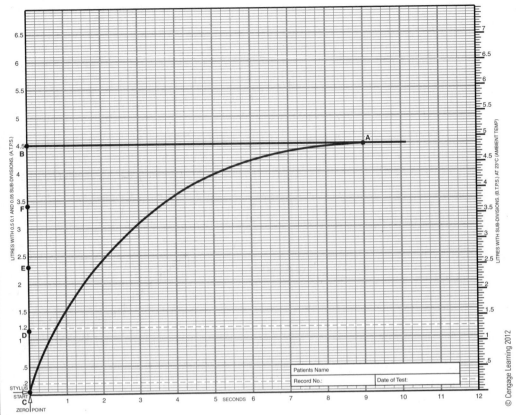

Figure 2-20 Determining the FVC and the four 25% segments of the FVC tracing.

© Cengage Learning 2012

Figure 2-20   Step 1. From the PFT tracing, locate the highest point at the end of the tracing (point A).
Step 2. From point A, draw a horizontal line until it intersects the volume (y) axis (point B).
Step 3. The difference between point B and the starting point C (4.5 L) represents the FVC.
Step 4. Divide the 4.5 L by 4 to obtain four equal segments. Plot the points D, E, F on the volume (y) axis to divide segment BC into four equal segments. The volume between points C and D represents the first 25% of the volume expired during the FVC maneuver. The volume between points D and F represents the middle 50% of the expired volume. The volume between points B and F represents the last 25% of the expired volume.

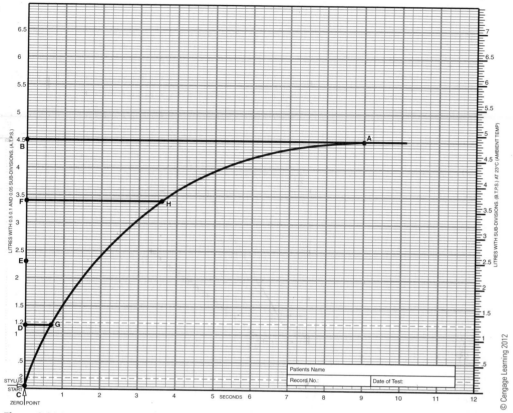

Figure 2-21 Determining the middle 50% of FVC on the graph paper (points D, F) and the spirograph (points G, H).

Figure 2-21   Step 5. From point D, draw a horizontal line until it intersects the PFT tracing (point G). Do the same from point F until the line intersects the PFT tracing (point H).

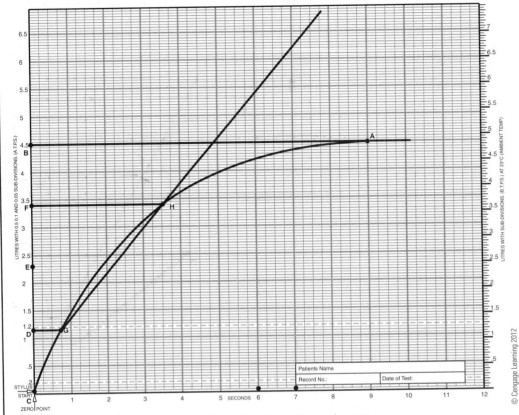

Figure 2-22 Determining the slope of the spirograph tracing on the graph paper.

Figure 2-22   Step 6. Use a ruler to draw a straight line joining points G and H. Extend this straight line to the top of the graph paper. This is the flow slope for this FEF$_{25-75\%}$ determination.

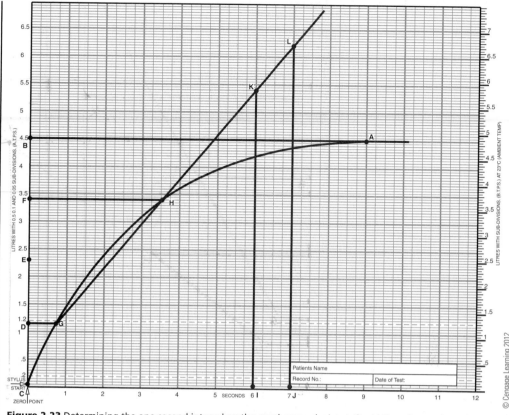

Figure 2-23 Determining the one-second interval on the graph paper (points I, J) and the spirograph tracing (points K, L).

Figure 2-23   Step 7. Along the time (x) axis, select two adjacent second-lines and mark them points I and J. In the example shown, the 6th and 7th second-lines are used. One may wish to use two other adjacent second-lines as long as the resulting drawings do not overlap or become too close to other existing lines. The result would be identical because any two adjacent lines intersect the same slope.

Step 8. From point I, follow the second-line vertically until it intersects the slope (point K). Do the same from point J until it intersects the slope (point L).

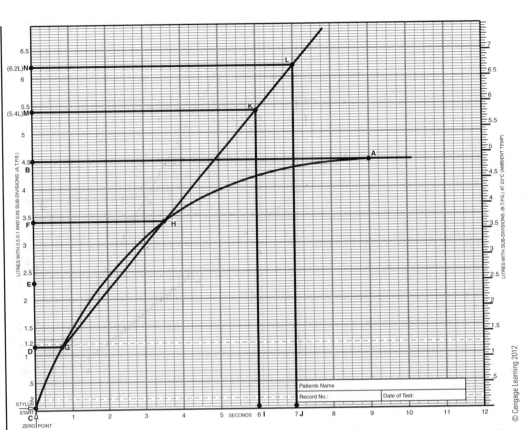

Figure 2-24 Determining the volume (L) that corresponds to the one-second interval (sec) on the slope. The unit of this reading is L/sec.

Figure 2-24   Step 9. From point K, draw a horizontal line until it intersects the volume (y) axis (point M). Do the same from point L until it intersects the volume (y) axis (point N). Step 10. The difference between the volume readings taken at points N and M represents the flow rate of the middle 50% of volume expired during the FVC maneuver.

$$\text{FEF}_{25-75\%} = (6.2\ L - 5.4\ L)/\text{sec}$$
$$= 0.8\ L/\text{sec}$$

EXERCISE   From the PFT tracing (Figure 2-25), find FEF$_{25-75\%}$.

[Answer: FEF$_{25-75\%}$ = (6.3 L − 5.25 L)/sec or 1.05 L/sec] (See Figure 2-26.)

REFERENCE   Ruppel

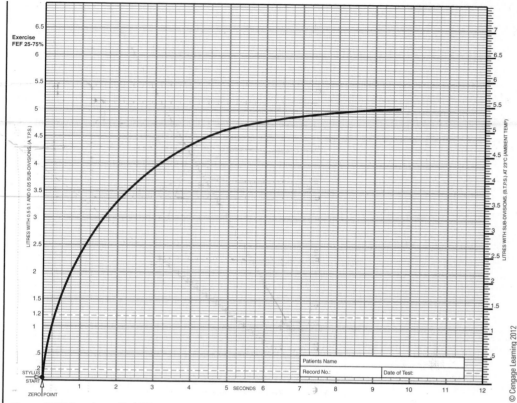

Figure 2-25 Exercise to find FEF$_{25-75\%}$.

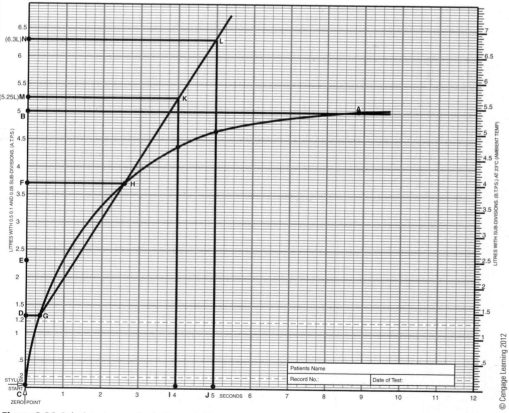

Figure 2-26 Solutions to exercise in Figure 2-25.

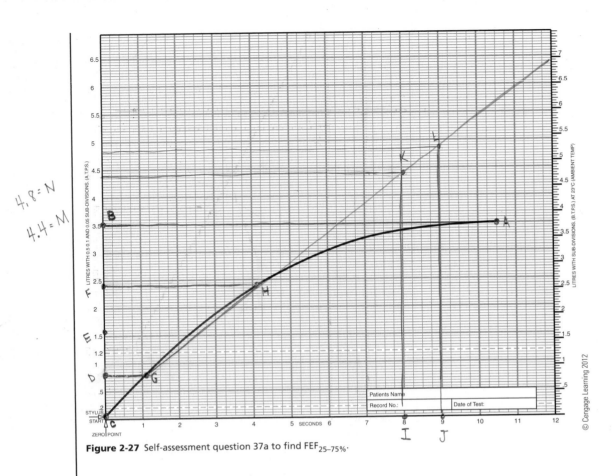

4,8 = N

4.4 = M

Figure 2-27 Self-assessment question 37a to find FEF$_{25-75\%}$.

© Cengage Learning 2012

SELF-ASSESSMENT QUESTIONS

37a. From the PFT tracing (Figure 2-27), find FEF$_{25-75\%}$.

4.8 - 4.4 = .4

FEF$_{25-75\%}$ = .4

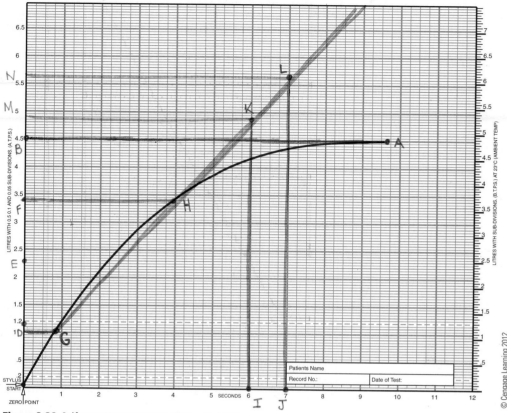

Figure 2-28 Self-assessment question 37b to find FEF$_{25-75\%}$.

37b. From the PFT tracing (Figure 2-28), find FEF$_{25-75\%}$.

$$5.7 - 4.8 = .9$$

$$FEF_{25-75\%} = .9$$

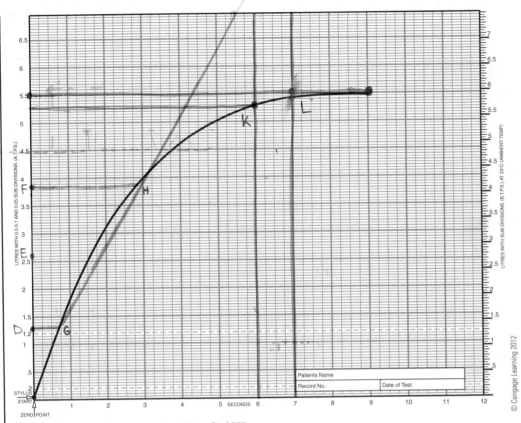

Figure 2-29 Self-assessment question 37c to find FEF$_{25-75\%}$.

37c. From the PFT tracing (Figure 2-29), find FEF$_{25-75\%}$.

$$\begin{array}{r} 1.375 \\ 1.3 \\ \hline 2.6 \\ 1.3 \\ \hline 3.9 \end{array}$$

$$5.3 - 5.5 = .2$$

$$FEF_{25-75\%} = .2$$

Chapter

38

Gas Law Equations

NOTES

Boyle's law (Robert Boyle)

Pressure and volume are inversely related. For example, a diver upon ascending to the surface (decreasing barometric pressure) must exhale more than he inhales to get a rid of the increasing lung volume. In respiratory care, this relationship between pressure and volume can be used to measure indirectly the functional residual capacity or the residual volume.

Charles' law (Jacques Charles)

The volume and absolute temperature (in kelvins) are directly related. Charles' law is most commonly used in respiratory care to correct lung volumes and flow rates measured at room temperature to that measured at body temperature.**

Gay-Lussac's law (Joseph Gay-Lussac)

The pressure and temperature are directly related. For example, the air pressure in a car tire increases as the surrounding temperature increases, and vice versa.

Combined Gas Law

This is also called the modified Ideal Gas Law. The Combined Gas Law accounts for all three factors (P, V, T) affecting gas behaviors. This equation is especially useful when precise measurements are required.

EQUATION 1   Boyle's law: $P_1 \times V_1 = P_2 \times V_2$ (Temperature is constant)

EQUATION 2   Charles' law: $\dfrac{V_1}{T_1} = \dfrac{V_2}{T_2}$ (Pressure is constant)

EQUATION 3   Gay-Lussac's Law: $\dfrac{P_1}{T_1} = \dfrac{P_2}{T_2}$ (Volume is constant)

EQUATION 4   Combined Gas Law: $\dfrac{P_1 \times V_1}{T_1} = \dfrac{P_2 \times V_2}{T_2}$

P : Barometric pressure in mm Hg
V : Volume in mL
T : Temperature in kelvins*
1 : Original values
2 : New values

EXAMPLE   See: Gas Volume Corrections.

EXERCISE

$P_1 \times V_1 = P_2 \times V_2$ is the _____ law.

$\dfrac{P_1}{T_1} = \dfrac{P_2}{T_2}$ is the _____ law.

$\dfrac{V_1}{T_1} = \dfrac{V_2}{T_2}$ is the _____ law.

Write the Combined Gas Law equation: _____

_____

[Answer: Boyle's; Gay-Lussac's; Charles'; $\dfrac{P_1 V_1}{T_1} = \dfrac{P_2 V_2}{T_2}$]

REFERENCE   Wilkins (2)

SEE   *Gas Volume Corrections.*

*See: Temperature Conversion (°C to K)

**ATPS to BTPS

SELF-ASSESSMENT QUESTIONS

MATCHING: Match the gas laws with the respective equations. Use only *three* of the answers in Column II.

Column I **Column II**

38a. Gay-Lussac's law (A) $P_1 V_1 = P_2 V_2$

38b. Charles' law (B) $\dfrac{P_1}{V_1} = \dfrac{P_2}{V_2}$

38c. Boyle's law (C) $\dfrac{V_1}{T_1} = \dfrac{V_2}{T_2}$

(D) $\dfrac{P_1}{T_1} = \dfrac{P_2}{T_2}$

38d. $P_1 \times V_1 = P_2 \times V_2$ is which of the following gas laws?

    (A) Gay-Lussac's

    (B) Charles'

    (C) Boyle's

    (D) Combined

38e. Charles' law is represented by the equation:

    (A) $P_1 \times V_1 = P_2 \times V_2$

    (B) $\dfrac{P_1}{T_1} = \dfrac{P_2}{T_2}$

    (C) $\dfrac{V_1}{T_1} = \dfrac{V_2}{T_2}$

    (D) $\dfrac{P_1}{V_1} = \dfrac{P_2}{V_2}$

38f. Gay-Lussac's law is represented by the equation:

    (A) $P_1 \times V_1 = P_2 \times V_2$

    (B) $\dfrac{P_1}{T_1} = \dfrac{P_2}{T_2}$

    (C) $\dfrac{V_1}{T_1} = \dfrac{V_2}{T_2}$

    (D) $\dfrac{P_1}{V_1} = \dfrac{P_2}{V_2}$

38g. According to Charles' law, at constant _____, the gas volume varies directly with the _____.

    (A) pressure; diffusion rate

    (B) temperature; pressure

    (C) pressure; temperature

    (D) temperature; solubility

38h. Correction of lung volumes and flow rates from ATPS to BTPS is based on:

   (A) Gay-Lussac's law.
   (B) Charles' law.
   (C) Boyle's law.
   (D) Bohr effect.

38i. In using the gas law equations, the temperature must first be converted to:

   (A) degrees Celsius.
   (B) degrees Fahrenheit.
   (C) kelvins.
   (D) degrees Centigrade.

38j. Which gas law states that at a constant temperature the gas volume varies inversely with the pressure?

   (A) Charles' law
   (B) Dalton's law
   (C) Boyle's law
   (D) Ideal Gas Law

Chapter

39

Gas Volume Corrections

NOTES

Before using these equations for gas volume corrections, the temperature must be converted to the Kelvin (K) temperature scale.

For gas volume correction problems involving *dry gas*, delete P_{H_2O} and use only P_B.

For gas correction problems involving the same pressure, delete P_1 and P_2 from the Combined Gas Law equation, and it becomes:

> Charles' law: $\dfrac{V_1}{T_1} = \dfrac{V_2}{T_2}$

To find new volume (V_2) or new temperature (T_2):

> $V_2 = \dfrac{V_1 \times T_2}{T_1}$ or $T_2 = \dfrac{V_2 \times T_1}{V_1}$

For gas correction problems involving the same temperature, delete T_1 and T_2 from the Combined Gas Law equation, and it becomes:

> Boyle's law: $P_1 \times V_1 = P_2 \times V_2$

To find new volume (V_2) or new pressure (P_2):

> $V_2 = \dfrac{P_1 \times V_1}{P_2}$ or $P_2 = \dfrac{P_1 \times V_1}{V_2}$

For gas correction problems involving the same volume, delete V_1 and V_2 from the Combined Gas Law equation, and it becomes:

> Gay-Lussac's law: $\dfrac{P_1}{T_1} = \dfrac{P_2}{T_2}$

EQUATION

Since $\dfrac{P_1 \times V_1}{T_1} = \dfrac{P_2 \times V_2}{T_2}$ (Combined Gas Law).

$$V_2 = \frac{P_1 \times V_1 \times T_2}{T_1 \times P_2}$$

V_2 : New gas volume in mL
P_1 : Original pressure ($P_B - P_{H_2O}$)
V_1 : Original gas volume in mL
T_2 : New temperature in kelvins (K)
T_1 : Original temperature in kelvins (K)
P_2 : New pressure ($P_B - P_{H_2O}$)

EXAMPLE 1

Given: 100 mL of saturated gas volume measured at 25°C and 750 mm Hg.

Find the new saturated gas volume measured at 37°C and 760 mm Hg.

At 25°C, $P_{H_2O} = 23.8$ mm Hg (Appendix R).
$P_1 = P_B1 - P_{H_2O} = (750 - 23.8)$ mm Hg $= 726.2$ mm Hg
At 37°C, $P_{H_2O} = 47$ mm Hg (Appendix R).
$P_2 = P_B2 - P_{H_2O} = (760 - 47)$ mm Hg $= 713$ mm Hg
$V_1 = 100$ mL
$T_1 = 25°C = (25 + 273)K = 298$ K
$T_2 = 37°C = (37 + 273)K = 310$ K

$$V_2 = \frac{P_1 \times V_1 \times T_2}{T_1 \times P_2}$$

$$= \frac{726.2 \times 100 \times 310}{298 \times 713}$$

$$= \frac{22,512,200}{212,474}$$

$$= 105.95 \text{ or } 106 \text{ mL}$$

EXAMPLE 2

A saturated tidal volume of 500 mL was measured at 24°C and 750 mm Hg. Find the new saturated gas volume corrected to 37°C and 760 mm Hg.
Given: At 24°C, $P_{H_2O} = 22.4$ mm Hg (Appendix R)

At 37°C, $P_{H_2O} = 47$ mm Hg (Appendix R)

NOTES (continued)

To find new pressure (P_2) or new temperature (T_2):

$$P_2 = \frac{P_1 \times T_2}{T_1} \quad \text{or} \quad T_2 = \frac{P_2 \times T_1}{P_1}$$

Since at 24°C, $P_{H_2O} = 22.4$ mm Hg,

$P_1 = P_B1 - P_{H_2O} = (750 - 22.4)$ mm Hg $= 727.6$ mm Hg

Since at 37°C, $P_{H_2O} = 47$ mm Hg,

$P_2 = P_B2 - P_{H_2O} = (760 - 47)$ mm Hg $= 713$ mm Hg

$V_1 = 500$ mL

$T_1 = 24°C = (24 + 273)K = 297$ K

$T_2 = 37°C = (37 + 273)K = 310$ K

$$V_2 = \frac{P_1 \times V_1 \times T_2}{T_1 \times P_2}$$

$$= \frac{727.6 \times 500 \times 310}{297 \times 713}$$

$$= \frac{112,778,000}{211,761}$$

$$= 532.6 \text{ or } 533 \text{ mL}$$

EXERCISE 1

Given: 100 mL of dry gas volume measured at 28°C and 760 mm Hg. Find the dry gas volume measured at 37°C and 760 mm Hg.

[Answer: $P_1 = 760$ mm Hg $P_2 = 760$ mm Hg
  $T_1 = 301$ K $T_2 = 310$ K
  $V_1 = 100$ mL $V_2 = 102.99$ or 103 mL]

EXERCISE 2

A saturated total lung capacity (*TLC*) of 2,500 mL was measured at 27°C and 755 mm Hg. Find the new saturated *TLC* corrected to 37°C and 758 mm Hg.
Given: At 27°C, P_{H_2O} = 26.7 mm Hg
       At 37°C, P_{H_2O} = 47 mm Hg

[Answer: $P_1 = 728.3$ mm Hg $P_2 = 711$ mm Hg
  $T_1 = 300$ K $T_2 = 310$ K
  $V_1 = 2,500$ mL $V_2 = 2,646$ mL]

REFERENCE

Wilkins (2)

SEE

Temperature Conversion (°C to K).

SELF-ASSESSMENT QUESTIONS

39a. Given:

$P_1 = 760$ mm Hg $P_2 = 755$ mm Hg

$T_1 = 300$ K $T_2 = 310$ K

$V_1 = 800$ mL

Find V_2 using the Combined Gas Law.

(A) 809 mL

(B) 814 mL

(C) 825 mL

(D) 832 mL

$V_1 = 1,000 \, mL$

$T_1 = 28°C$

$P_1 = 750 \, mm \, Hg$

$V_2 = ?$

$T_2 = 37°C$

$P_2 = 760 \, mm \, Hg$

39b. A saturated gas sample of 1,000 mL was measured at 28°C and 750 mm Hg. Find the new saturated gas volume corrected to 37°C and 760 mm Hg. (At 28°C, $P_{H_2O} = 28.3$ mm Hg; at 37°C, $P_{H_2O} = 47$ mm Hg.)

(A) 1,042 mL

(B) 1,016 mL

(C) 995 mL

(D) 987 mL

39c. The forced vital capacity (*FVC*) of a patient measured at 26°C and 760 mm Hg is 3,000 mL. Find the new *FVC* corrected to 37°C and 758 mm Hg. (At 26°C, $P_{H_2O} = 25.2$ mm Hg; at 37°C, $P_{H_2O} = 47$ mm Hg.)

(A) 3,119 mL

(B) 3,161 mL

(C) 3,203 mL

(D) 3,215 mL

39d. Given the following information: measured tidal volume (V_T) = 670 mL; temperature and pressure under which V_T was obtained = 27°C and 758 mm Hg. Calculate the corrected V_T at 37°C and 760 mm Hg. (At 27°C, $P_{H_2O} = 26.7$ mm Hg; at 37°C, $P_{H_2O} = 47$ mm Hg.)

(A) 665 mL

(B) 680 mL

(C) 691 mL

(D) 710 mL

Chapter

40

Graham's Law
of Diffusion Coefficient

NOTES

In 1833, the Scottish inorganic and physical chemist Thomas Graham proposed Graham's law, which states that the rate of gas diffusion is inversely proportional to the square root of its gram molecular weight. The solubility coefficient in the equation is added for calculation of the diffusion coefficient.

In pulmonary disorders that impair the lung's diffusion rate, hypoxia is usually a more difficult situation to correct than is hypercapnia because of the low diffusion coefficient of oxygen.

EQUATION

$$D = \frac{\text{Sol. Coeff.}}{\sqrt{\text{gmw}}}$$

D : Diffusion coefficient

Sol. Coeff. : Solubility coefficient of gas

$\sqrt{gmw}$: Square root of gram molecular weight of gas

EXAMPLE

The diffusion coefficient of carbon dioxide is 19 times $\left(\dfrac{0.077}{0.004}\right)$ greater than that of oxygen. This is shown by computing the diffusion coefficient of each gas.

$$D_{\text{carbon dioxide}} = \frac{0.510}{\sqrt{44}} \quad D_{\text{oxygen}} = \frac{0.023}{\sqrt{32}}$$

$$= \frac{0.510}{6.633} \qquad\qquad = \frac{0.023}{5.657}$$

$$= 0.077 \qquad\qquad\quad = 0.004$$

The difference in diffusion coefficient between carbon dioxide and oxygen explains why a small carbon dioxide pressure gradient of 6 mm Hg ($P_{\bar{v}}CO_2$ 46 mm Hg $- P_A CO_2$ 40 mm Hg) across the alveolar-capillary membrane is sufficient for carbon dioxide elimination. On the other hand, a much larger pressure gradient of 60 mm Hg ($P_A O_2$ 100 mm Hg $- P_{\bar{v}}O_2$ 40 mm Hg) is needed for oxygen uptake by the pulmonary capillaries.

REFERENCES

Wilkins (2)

SEE

Fick's Law of Diffusion.

SELF-ASSESSMENT QUESTIONS

40a. The diffusion coefficient of a gas is described by:

(A) Charles' law.
(B) Gay-Lussac's law.
(C) Graham's law.
(D) Henry's law.

40b. The diffusion coefficient of a gas is _____ related to its solubility coefficient and _____ related to the square root of its gram molecular weight.

(A) directly; inversely
(B) directly; directly
(C) inversely; inversely
(D) inversely; directly

40c. The diffusion coefficient of carbon dioxide is about _____ times higher than that of oxygen. For this reason, hypoxia is _____ to treat than hypercapnia in the absence of airway obstruction.

(A) 30; more difficult
(B) 30; easier
(C) 19; easier
(D) 19; more difficult

Chapter

41

Helium/Oxygen (He/O$_2$) Flow Rate Conversion

NOTES

A conversion factor (e.g., 1.8 or 1.6) must be used if an oxygen flow meter is used to regulate a helium/oxygen gas mixture. This factor provides a more accurate flow rate because of the lower density of a helium/oxygen mixture.

The conversion factors are 1.8 for an 80%He/20%O$_2$ mixture and 1.6 for a 70%He/30%O$_2$ mixture.

Helium/oxygen mixture is sometimes used in patients with diffuse airway obstruction or obstruction caused by excessive secretions. It provides relief from hypoxia because a helium/oxygen mixture has a higher diffusion rate than oxygen or air alone.

Because of the high diffusion rate of a helium/oxygen mixture, a closely fitted oxygen delivering device such as a nonrebreathing mask should be used.

EQUATION 1

Actual flow rate of 80%He/20%O$_2$ = Flow rate × 1.8

EQUATION 2

Actual flow rate of 70%He/30%O$_2$ = Flow rate × 1.6

EXAMPLE

Given: A gas mixture of 70%He/30%O$_2$ is running at a flow rate of 10 L/min with an oxygen flow meter. What is the actual flow rate of this He/O$_2$ gas mixture?

Actual flow rate of 70%He/30%O$_2$ = Flow rate × 1.6
= 10 L/min × 1.6
= 16 L/min

EXERCISE

Given: An oxygen flow meter is being used to administer 8 L/min of an 80%He/20%O$_2$ gas mixture. What is the actual flow rate of this gas mixture?

[Answer: Flow rate = 14.4 L/min]

REFERENCE

Wilkins (2)

SELF-ASSESSMENT QUESTIONS

41a. Given: a gas mixture of 70%He/30%O$_2$ is running at a flow rate of 5 L/min on an oxygen flow meter. What is the actual flow rate of this gas mixture?

(A) 4 L/min
(B) 6 L/min
(C) 7 L/min
(D) 8 L/min

41b. An oxygen flow meter is being used to regulate a gas mixture of 70%He/30%O$_2$. If the flow rate is set at 6 L/min, what is the actual flow rate of this He/O$_2$ gas mixture?

(A) 12 L/min
(B) 10.8 L/min
(C) 9.6 L/min
(D) 8.3 L/min

41c. Calculate the actual flow rate if an 80%He/20%O$_2$ gas mixture is running at 5 L/min on an oxygen flow meter.

(A) 6 L/min

(B) 7 L/min

(C) 8 L/min

(D) 9 L/min

41d. If an oxygen flow meter is used to regulate an 80%He/20%O$_2$ gas mixture and a flow rate of 10 L/min is desired, what should be the flow rate set on the oxygen flow meter?

(A) 4.5 L/min

(B) 5.6 L/min

(C) 6.3 L/min

(D) 7.7 L/min

Chapter

42

Humidity Deficit

In the humidity deficit equation, 43.9 mg/L represents the maximum humidity capacity at body temperature. Humidity deficit is dependent on the humidity content of the inspired air. A higher humidity content in the inspired air gives a lower humidity deficit. On the other hand, a lower humidity content means a higher humidity deficit.

Humidifiers and aerosol nebulizers are used to increase the humidity content of the inspired air, and thus, a lower humidity deficit.

EQUATION

HD = Capacity − Content
HD   :   Humidity deficit in mg/L
Capacity   :   Maximum amount of water the alveolar air can hold at body temperature (43.9 mg/L at 37°C). Also known as maximum absolute humidity
Content   :   Humidity content of inspired air; actual humidity or absolute humidity

EXAMPLE

Calculate the humidity deficit at body temperature if the inspired air has a humidity content of 26 mg/L. The humidity capacity at body temperature is 43.9 mg/L (Appendix R).
HD = Capacity − Content
    = 43.9 − 26
    = 17.9 or 18 mg/L

EXERCISE 1

Calculate the humidity deficit if the humidity content is 34 mg/L and capacity is 43.9 mg/L.

[Answer: HD = 9.9 or 10 mg/L]

EXERCISE 2

Use Appendix R to find the humidity capacity at normal body temperature (37°C) and calculate the humidity deficit when the inspired air has a humidity content of 32 mg/L.

[Answer: HD = 11.9 or 12 mg/L]

REFERENCE

Wilkins (1)

SEE

Appendix R: Humidity Capacity of Saturated Gas at Selected Temperatures.

SELF-ASSESSMENT QUESTIONS

42a. What is the humidity deficit at body temperature if the humidity content of inspired air is 22 mg/L? (Humidity capacity at 37°C = 43.9 mg/L.)

(A) 11 mg/L
(B) 22 mg/L
(C) 30 mg/L
(D) 37 mg/L

42b. Calculate the humidity deficit at body temperature if the inspired air has a humidity content of 27 mg/L and the humidity capacity at 37°C is 43.9 mg/L.

(A) 17 mg/L
(B) 27 mg/L
(C) 32 mg/L
(D) 37 mg/L

42c. Which of the following is the most effective device to reduce the humidity deficit?

(A) Heat and moisture exchanger
(B) Continuous cool aerosol
(C) Continuous heated aerosol
(D) Humidifier

Chapter

43

I:E Ratio

See Exercise 1 for reserve *I:E* ratio.

NOTE

When the inspiratory time is *longer* than the expiratory time, divide both *I* time and *E* time by the expiratory time to get a reverse *I:E* ratio.

$$I : E = \left(\frac{I \text{ time}}{E \text{ time}} \right) : \left(\frac{E \text{ time}}{E \text{ time}} \right)$$

EXAMPLE 1

When the *I* time and *E* time are known:

What is the *I:E* ratio if the inspiratory time is 0.4 sec and the expiratory time is 1.2 sec?

$$I : E = \left(\frac{I \text{ time}}{I \text{ time}} \right) : \left(\frac{E \text{ time}}{I \text{ time}} \right)$$

$$= \left(\frac{0.4}{0.4} \right) : \left(\frac{1.2}{0.4} \right)$$

$$= \quad 1 \quad : \quad 3$$

EXERCISE 1

What is the *I:E* ratio if the inspiratory time is 0.6 sec and the expiratory time is 0.4 sec?

[Answer: *I:E* = 1.5 : 1]

EXAMPLE 2

When the *I* time % is known:

What is the *I:E* ratio if the inspiratory time ratio is 25% or 0.25?

$$I : E = \left(\frac{I \text{ time \%}}{I \text{ time \%}} \right) : \left(\frac{1 - I \text{ time \%}}{I \text{ time \%}} \right)$$

$$= \left(\frac{0.25}{0.25} \right) : \left(\frac{1 - 0.25}{0.25} \right)$$

$$= \quad 1 \quad : \left(\frac{0.75}{0.25} \right)$$

$$= \quad 1 \quad : \quad 3$$

EXERCISE 2

What is the *I:E* ratio if the inspiratory time ratio is 33% or 0.33?

[Answer: *I:E* = 1 : 2]

EXAMPLE 3

When the *I* time and *f* are known:

What is the *I:E* ratio if the inspiratory time is 1.5 sec and the frequency is 15/min?

I time = 1.5 sec

$$E \text{ time} = \frac{60}{f} - I \text{ time}$$
$$= \frac{60}{15} - 1.5$$
$$= 4 - 1.5$$
$$= 2.5 \text{ sec}$$

$$I : E = I \text{ time}: E \text{ time}$$
$$= 1.5 : 2.5$$
$$= \left(\frac{1.5}{1.5}\right) : \left(\frac{2.5}{1.5}\right)$$
$$= 1 : 1.67$$

EXERCISE 3

What is the *I:E* ratio if the inspiratory time is 0.6 sec and the frequency is 20/min?

[Answer: *I:E* = 1 : 4]

EXAMPLE 4

When the minute volume ($\dot{V}_E$) and flow rate are known:

Given: V_T = 800 mL (0.8 L)
      f = 12/min
      Flow rate = 40 L/min

What is the *I:E* ratio?

$I:E$ ratio = (Minute volume) : (Flow rate − Minute volume)
$= (V_T \times f)$: (Flow rate − $V_T \times f$)
$= (0.8 \times 12) : (40 - 0.8 \times 12)$
$= 9.6 : (40 - 9.6)$
$= 9.6 : 30.4$
[divide both sides of this ratio by 9.6]
$= 1 : 3.2$

EXERCISE 4

Given: V_T = 1,000 mL (1 L)
      f = 10/min
      Flow rate = 50 L/min
What is the *I:E* ratio?

[Answer: *I:E* = 1 : 4]

SELF-ASSESSMENT QUESTIONS

43a. Calculate the *I:E* ratio if the inspiratory time is 0.4 sec and the expiratory time is 0.6 sec.

(A) 1.5 : 1
(B) 1 : 1
(C) 1 : 1.5
(D) 1 : 2

43b. What is the *I:E* ratio if the inspiratory time is 0.5 sec and the expiratory time is 1.5 sec?

(A) 1 : 1
(B) 1 : 2
(C) 1 : 3
(D) 2 : 1

$$\frac{0.5}{0.5} : \frac{1.5}{0.5} \quad = 1:3$$

43c. Calculate the *I:E* ratio when the inspiratory time is 1.2 sec and the expiratory time is 1.8 sec.

(A) 1 : 1.5
(B) 1 : 2
(C) 1 : 2.5
(D) 1 : 3

$$\frac{I}{I} : \frac{E}{I} \qquad \frac{1.2}{1.2} : \frac{1.8}{1.2} = 1:1.5$$

43d. Which of the following sets of inspiratory time (*I* time) and expiratory time (*E* time) does not equal an *I:E* ratio of 1:2?

	I time (sec)	*E* time (sec)
(A)	2.0	4.0
(B)	1.5	3.0
(C)	0.8	1.6
(D)	2.0	1.0

43e. Calculate the *I:E* ratio when the inspiratory time ratio is 25%.

(A) 1 : 3
(B) 1 : 4
(C) 1 : 5
(D) 4 : 1

$$\left(\frac{0.25}{0.25}\right) : \left(\frac{1-0.25}{0.25}\right)$$

$$1 : 3$$

43f. What is the *I:E* ratio if the inspiratory time ratio is 40% or 0.4?

(A) 1 : 1.5
(B) 1 : 2
(C) 1 : 2.5
(D) 1 : 3

$$\frac{(0.40)}{(0.40)} : \frac{(1-0.40)}{0.40} = 1:1.5$$

43g. The inspiratory time is set at 30% of one complete respiratory cycle. The *I:E* ratio is about:

(A) 1 : 0.3
(B) 1 : 0.7
(C) 1 : 1.3
(D) 1 : 2.3

$$\frac{(0.30)}{(0.30)} : \frac{(1-0.30)}{(0.30)} = 1:2.3$$

43h. Calculate the *I:E* ratio when the inspiratory time on a ventilator is set at 20% of one complete respiratory cycle.

(A) 1 : 1
(B) 1 : 2
(C) 1 : 3
(D) 1 : 4

$$\frac{0.20}{0.20} : \frac{1-0.20}{0.20} =$$

$$1:4$$

43i. Which of the following inspiratory time percent (%) settings would give an *I:E* ratio of 1:3?

(A) 10%
(B) 20%
(C) 25%
(D) 30%

43j. What is the *I:E* ratio if the inspiratory time is 0.5 sec and the frequency is 30/min?

(A) 1 : 3
(B) 1 : 4
(C) 1 : 5
(D) 4 : 1

43k. Calculate the *I:E* ratio for the following settings: inspiratory time = 1 sec frequency = 20/min

(A) 1 : 1
(B) 1 : 2
(C) 1 : 3
(D) 1 : 4

43l. Given: inspiratory time = 1.5 sec frequency = 16/min. Find the expiratory time. What is the *I:E* ratio at these settings?

(A) 0.75 sec; 1 : 0.5
(B) 1.5 sec; 1 : 1
(C) 2.25 sec; 1 : 1.5
(D) 2.63 sec; 1 : 1.75

43m. A patient on a ventilator has an inspiratory time of 1.2 sec and a ventilator frequency of 25/min. What are the expiratory time and *I:E* ratio at these settings?

(A) 0.96 sec; 1 : 0.8
(B) 1.2 sec; 1 : 1
(C) 1.44 sec; 1 : 1.2
(D) 1.68 sec; 1 : 1.4

43n. Which of the following settings would *not* provide an *I:E* ratio of about 1: 0.5?

	I time (sec)	*f*
(A)	2.0	20
(B)	1.6	25
(C)	1.33	30
(D)	3	15

43o. Given: V_T = 1,000 mL (1 L), f = 10/min, flow rate = 40 L/min. What is the *I:E* ratio?

(A) 1 : 3
(B) 1 : 4
(C) 1 : 5
(D) 4 : 1

43p. Given: $V_T = 1,000$ mL (1 L), $f = 12$/min flow rate $= 50$ L/min.
    What is the calculated I:E ratio?

(A) 1 : 3.2
(B) 1 : 2.8
(C) 1 : 2.4
(D) 1 : 2

43q. Which of the following settings has a calculated I:E ratio of 1 : 4?

	V_T (mL)	f	Flow rate
(A)	800	15	40
(B)	800	15	45
(C)	800	15	50
(D)	800	15	60

43r. A patient on the ventilator has a tidal volume of 850 mL (0.85 L),
    frequency of 16/min, and flow rate of 50 L/min. Based on these
    settings, what is the I:E ratio? If the flow rate is increased to
    60 L/min, will the E ratio be longer or shorter?

(A) 1 : 2.7; E ratio will be longer (3.4)
(B) 1 : 2.7; E ratio will be shorter (2.0)
(C) 1 : 2.4; E ratio will be shorter (1.7)
(D) 1 : 2.1; E ratio will be shorter (1.4)

43s. A patient has the following settings on a mechanical ventilator:
    $V_T = 750$ mL (0.75 L), $f = 16$/min, flow rate $= 50$ L/min.
    Calculate the I:E ratio based on these settings. If a *longer* E ratio
    is desired, should the flow rate be increased or decreased?

(A) 1 : 1.6; flow rate should be increased
(B) 1 : 2.4; flow rate should be increased
(C) 1 : 2.4; flow rate should be decreased
(D) 1 : 3.2; flow rate should be increased

43t. The following settings are found on a mechanical ventilator:
    $V_T = 900$ mL (0.9 L), $f = 14$/min, flow rate $= 55$ L/min. What is
    the calculated I:E ratio based on these settings? If a *shorter*
    E ratio is desired, what should be done to the flow rate?

(A) 1 : 3.1; flow rate should be increased
(B) 1 : 3.1; flow rate should be decreased
(C) 1 : 3.4; flow rate should be increased
(D) 1 : 3.4; flow rate should be decreased

43u. An I:E ratio of 1.5:1 is the same as:

(A) 1 : 0.5
(B) 1 : 0.67
(C) 1 : 0.8
(D) 1 : 1.5

Chapter

44

Law of LaPlace

NOTE
This equation illustrates two important concepts in respiratory care—one physiological and the other pathophysiological.

EQUATION

$$P = \frac{2ST}{r}$$

P : Pressure in dynes/cm^2
ST : Surface tension in dyne/cm
r : Radius in cm

Physiological consideration
In normal human lungs there are millions of alveoli varying in sizes. If the surface tensions in these alveoli were identical, the smaller alveoli would empty into the larger alveoli [because low radius (r) means a high pressure (P) at constant surface tension (ST)]. In reality, as normal alveoli decrease in size, the *relative* amount of surfactant increases, thus lowering the surface tension to maintain an equilibrium in the pressure gradient and stability of alveoli of varying sizes.

Pathophysiological consideration
The equation shows that the work of breathing (P) is directly related to the surface tension (ST) of the alveoli. Surfactant deficiency (as in premature lungs and ARDS) causes an increase in pulmonary surface tension, which in turn leads to an increase in the work of breathing. Atelectasis resulting from surfactant deficiency further hinders ventilation because of the inverse relationship between the size of the alveoli (r) and work of breathing (P).
Artificial and natural surfactants have been used successfully to reduce the surface tension of noncompliant lungs and to improve ventilation (e.g., surfactant deficiency in premature infants).

REFERENCE

Wilkins (2)

SELF-ASSESSMENT QUESTIONS

44a. In pulmonary physiology, _____ can be used to describe the relationship among work of breathing, surface tension, and size of alveoli.

(A) Law of LaPlace
(B) Dalton's law
(C) Henry's law
(D) Hooke's law

44b. If P in the Law of LaPlace represents work of breathing, it is directly related to the _____ and inversely related to the

_____.

(A) radius; surface tension
(B) surface tension; radius
(C) radius; partial pressure of gas
(D) surface tension; partial pressure of gas

44c. Based on the Law of LaPlace, alveolar units that become _____ cause _____ in the work of breathing.

(A) larger; an increase
(B) smaller; an increase
(C) smaller; a decrease
(D) smaller; no change

44d. Surfactant replacement therapy is effective in _____ the pulmonary surface tension and in _____ the work of breathing.

(A) increasing; decreasing
(B) increasing; increasing
(C) reducing; decreasing
(D) reducing; increasing

Chapter

45

Lung Volumes and Capacities

There are four lung volumes and four lung capacities. Lung volumes are distinct measurements that do not overlap each other. Lung capacities are measurements containing two or more lung volumes (Figure 2-30).

Residual volume, functional residual capacity, and total lung capacity cannot be measured directly. They must be measured by an indirect method such as helium dilution, nitrogen washout, body plethysmograph, or radiologic estimation.

Changes in lung volumes/ capacities may be used to distinguish restrictive and obstructive lung diseases. In general, restrictive lung diseases show decreases in lung volumes and capacities, whereas obstructive lung diseases have increases in residual volume. Functional residual capacity and total lung capacity may be increased in air trapping or hyperinflation of the lungs because residual volume is part of these two lung capacities (Figure 2-31).

EQUATION 1

$$TLC = IRV + V_T + ERV + RV$$
$$TLC = VC + RV$$
$$TLC = IC + FRC$$

EQUATION 2

$$VC = IRV + V_T + ERV$$
$$VC = IC + ERV$$
$$VC = TLC - RV$$

EQUATION 3

$$IC = IRV + V_T$$
$$IC = TLC - FRC$$
$$IC = VC - ERV$$

EQUATION 4

$$FRC = ERV + RV$$
$$FRC = TLC - IC$$

TLC : Total lung capacity
VC : Vital capacity
IC : Inspiratory capacity
FRC : Functional residual capacity
IRV : Inspiratory reserve volume
V_T : Tidal volume
ERV : Expiratory reserve volume
RV : Residual volume

NORMAL VALUES

Normal values depend on a person's gender, age, ethnic origin, height, weight, and smoking history. The traditional normal values for a young adult male are listed below to show calculation of lung volumes and capacities.

$TLC = 6,000$ mL; $VC = 4,800$ mL; $IC = 3,600$ mL;
$FRC = 2,400$ mL
$IRV = 3,100$ mL; $V_T = 500$ mL; $ERV = 1,200$ mL;
$RV = 1,200$ mL

EXAMPLE 1

What is the calculated residual volume if the total lung capacity is 5,800 mL and the vital capacity is 4,950 mL?

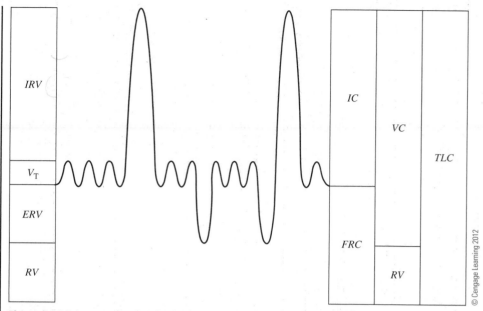

Figure 2-30 Spirogram showing the distribution of lung volumes and capacities.

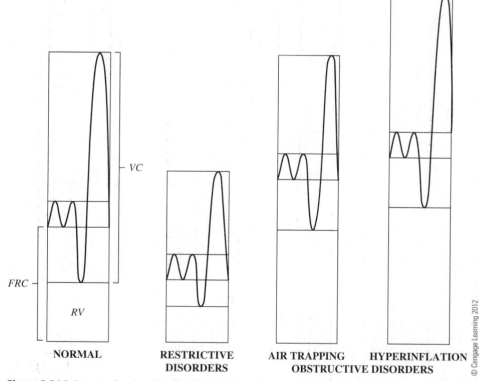

NORMAL   **RESTRICTIVE**   **AIR TRAPPING**   **HYPERINFLATION**
                    DISORDERS   **OBSTRUCTIVE DISORDERS**

Figure 2-31 Spirogram showing the alteration of lung volumes and capacities with restrictive and obstructive lung disorders.

$$TLC = VC + RV \text{ (equation 1)}$$
$$RV = TLC - VC$$
$$= 5,800 - 4,950$$
$$= 850 \text{ mL}$$

EXAMPLE 2

Given: Total lung capacity   =   6,400 mL
Functional residual capacity =   2,600 mL
What is the calculated inspiratory capacity?
$$IC = TLC - FRC \text{ (equation 3)}$$
$$= 6,400 - 2,600$$
$$= 3,800 \text{ mL}$$

EXERCISE 1

If the inspiratory capacity is 3,900 mL and the tidal volume is 620 mL, what is the calculated inspiratory reserve volume?

[Answer: IRV = 3,280 mL]

EXERCISE 2

Calculate the functional residual capacity if the expiratory reserve volume and residual volume are 1,100 mL and 1,500 mL, respectively.

[Answer: FRC = 2,600 mL]

EXERCISE 3

What is the calculated tidal volume if the inspiratory capacity is 3,450 mL and the inspiratory reserve volume is 2,950 mL?

[Answer: V_T = 500 mL]

REFERENCE

Ruppel

SEE

Appendix T, Lung Volumes, Capacities, and Ventilation.

SELF-ASSESSMENT QUESTIONS

45a. The sum of IRV and V_T is equal to:

(A) VC.
(B) TLC.
(C) IC.
(D) FRC.

45b. A patient's vital capacity can be calculated by the equation:

(A) $VC = IRV + ERV$.
(B) $VC = TLC - IRV$.
(C) $VC = IRV + V_T$.
(D) $VC = TLC - RV$.

45c. Which of the following cannot be measured directly by simple spirometry?

(A) RV

(B) V_T

(C) IRV

(D) ERV

45d. A patient's vital capacity can be calculated by using which of the following equations?

I. $TLC - RV = VC$

II. $IC + FRC = VC$

III. $IRV + V_T + ERV = VC$

IV. $FRC + V_T = VC$

V. $IC + ERV = VC$

(A) I, III, and V only

(B) II and IV only

(C) III and V only

(D) I, II, and IV only

45e. Which of the following equations cannot be used to calculate the total lung capacity (*TLC*)?

(A) $TLC = IRV + V_T + ERV + RV$

(B) $TLC = VC + RV$

(C) $TLC = IC + FRC$

(D) $TLC = IRV + V_T + ERV$

45f. Which of the following equations cannot be used to calculate the vital capacity (*VC*)?

(A) $VC = IRV + V_T$

(B) $VC = IRV + V_T + ERV$

(C) $VC = IC + ERV$

(D) $VC = IC + FRC - RV$

45g. All of the following equations are correct with the *exception* of:

(A) $IC = IRV + V_T$

(B) $VC = IC + FRC$

(C) $FRC = ERV + RV$

(D) $ERV = VC - IC$

MATCHING: Match the lung capacities with the values listed in Column II. Use only four answers from Column II.

Given: $IRV = 3{,}100$ mL, $V_T = 500$ mL, $ERV = 1{,}200$ mL, $RV = 1{,}200$ mL

Column I		Column II
45h.	VC	(A) 6,000 mL
45i.	FRC	(B) 4,800 mL
45j.	IC	(C) 3,600 mL
45k.	TLC	(D) 2,400 mL

45l. A pulmonary function study shows the following: $IRV =$ 1,200 mL, $V_T = 500$ mL, $ERV = 1,000$ mL. Based on these values, the patient's TLC is:

(A) 1,700 mL.

(B) 1,700 mL plus RV.

(C) 2,700 mL plus RV.

(D) 2,700 mL minus RV.

45m. Studies on a patient reveal the following: $IRV = 1,600$ mL, $V_T = 500$ mL, $ERV = 1,000$ mL. On the basis of these data, the patient's TLC is:

(A) 2,100 mL minus RV.

(B) 2,600 mL plus RV.

(C) 3,100 mL.

(D) 3,100 mL plus RV.

For questions 45n–q, use the following lung volumes to calculate the lung capacities for the next four questions:

$IRV = 3,000$ mL, $V_T = 650$ mL, $ERV = 1,100$ mL, $RV = 1,150$ mL

45n. Total lung capacity (TLC) is:

(A) 2,900 mL.

(B) 3,650 mL.

(C) 4,800 mL.

(D) 5,900 mL.

45o. Vital capacity (VC) is:

(A) 2,250 mL.

(B) 2,900 mL.

(C) 3,650 mL.

(D) 4,750 mL.

45p. Inspiratory capacity (IC) is:

(A) 2,250 mL.

(B) 2,900 mL.

(C) 3,650 mL.

(D) 4,750 mL.

45q. Functional residual capacity (FRC) is:

(A) 2,250 mL.

(B) 2,900 mL.

(C) 3,650 mL.

(D) 4,750 mL.

45r. Calculate the residual volume when the total lung capacity is
6,200 mL and the vital capacity is 4,900 mL.

(A) 1,100 mL
(B) 1,200 mL
(C) 1,300 mL
(D) 1,400 mL

44s. Given: total lung capacity = 5,500 mL, functional residual
capacity = 2,300 mL. What is the inspiratory capacity (*IC*)?

(A) 2,300 mL
(B) 3,200 mL
(C) 5,500 mL
(D) 7,800 mL

45t. If the inspiratory capacity is 3,200 mL and the tidal volume is
500 mL, what is the inspiratory reserve volume (*IRV*)?

(A) 500 mL
(B) 2,700 mL
(C) 3,200 mL
(D) 3,700 mL

Chapter

46

MDI/DPI Dosage

EQUATION

MDI/DPI Dosage = Dosage per inhalation × Number of inhalations

MDI/DPI Dosage : Dosage of drug delivered by a metered-dose inhaler or dry-powder inhaler

Dosage per inhalation: Determined by manufacturer

Number of inhalations: Prescribed by physician

EXAMPLE 1

A patient is using the DPI 250/50 Advair Diskus® BID. What is the total daily amount of prescribed medication for this patient?

Each inhalation of 250/50 Advair Diskus® provides 250 mcg of fluticasone and 50 mcg of salmeterol. As the patient is using this DPI inhaler two times per day, the daily dosage is calculated as follows:

$$
\begin{aligned}
\text{DPI Dosage} &= \text{(250 mcg of fluticasone and 50 mcg} \\
&\qquad \text{of salmeterol)} \times 2 \\
&= \text{500 mcg of fluticasone and 100 mcg} \\
&\qquad \text{of salmeterol}
\end{aligned}
$$

The total daily dosage is 500 mcg of fluticasone and 100 mcg of salmeterol.

EXAMPLE 2

The physician has written an order for Combivent® MDI 2 puffs QID and prn. The patient uses this inhaler six times in a 24-hour period. What is the total daily dosage?

Each inhalation of Combivent® contains 18 mcg of ipratropium bromide and 103 mcg of albuterol. The daily dosage can be calculated as follows:

$$
\begin{aligned}
\text{MDI Dosage} &= \text{(18 mcg of ipratropium and 103 mcg of} \\
&\qquad \text{albuterol)} \times 6 \times 2 \\
&= \text{(18 mcg of ipratropium and 103 mcg of} \\
&\qquad \text{albuterol)} \times 12 \\
&= \text{(216 mcg of ipratropium and 1,236 mcg} \\
&\qquad \text{of albuterol)}
\end{aligned}
$$

The total daily dosage is 216 mcg of ipratropium bromide and 1,236 mcg of albuterol sulfate.

EXERCISE 1   A patient uses eight puffs of Xopenex HFA® MDI in a 24-hour period. As each inhalation of this MDI provides 45 mcg of Xopenex®, what is the total daily dosage?

[Answer: MDI Dosage = 360 mcg]

EXAMPLE 2   The physician has ordered formoterol fumarate (Foradil Aerolizer®) BID for a patient. What is the total daily dosage? (Foradil provides 12 mcg per inhalation)

[Answer: DPI Dosage = 24 mcg]

REFERENCE   Colbert

SELF-ASSESSMENT QUESTIONS

46a. Each capsule of Spiriva® contains 18 mcg of tiotropium bromide. If the daily recommended frequency is once per day for patients 12 and older, what is the daily dosage?

(A) 18 mcg
(B) 36 mcg
(C) 180 mcg
(D) Insufficient information to calculate answer

46b. Two puffs of Serevent Diskus® provide how many mcg of salmeterol xinafoate? (Serevent Diskus® has 50 mcg/inhalation).

(A) 25 mcg
(B) 50 mcg
(C) 100 mcg
(D) Insufficient information to calculate answer

50 mcg x 2 puff = 100 mcg

46c. Two preparations of Symbicort® are available: 80/4.5 and 160/4.5. Which contains more formoterol per inhalation?

(A) 80/4.5
(B) 160/4.5
(C) Neither preparation contains formoterol.
(D) Both preparations contain the same amount of formoterol.

46d. The recommended starting total daily dose for flunisolide (Aerobid®) is 1 mg (1,000 mcg) each day to be given twice per day and 2 puffs each time. What is the dosage for each treatment consisting of 2 puffs?

(A) 0.25 mcg
(B) 500 mcg
(C) 250 mcg
(D) 2.5 mcg

46e. A patient has been using Maxair Autohaler® three times daily at 200 mcg per inhalation? What is the total daily dosage?

(A) 150 mcg
(B) 300 mcg
(C) 600 mcg
(D) 1,200 mcg

46f. For patients who are at least 12 years old, the recommended starting dose of mometasone furoate (Asmanex Twisthaler®) is 220 mcg each evening. The highest daily recommended dosage is 440 mcg. If a 110 mcg Asmanex DPI is available, how many inhalations should be used to obtain the starting dose and the highest daily dose?

(A) 1 inhalation for starting dose; 2 inhalations for highest dose
(B) 2 inhalations for starting dose; 4 inhalations for highest dose
(C) 2 inhalations for starting dose; 1 inhalation for highest dose
(D) 4 inhalations for starting dose; 2 inhalations for highest dose

Chapter

47

Mean Airway Pressure (*MAWP*)

NOTES

The mean airway pressure (*MAWP* or $\bar{P}aw$) is the average pressure in the airways over a series of breathing cycles, usually measured during mechanical ventilation.

MAWP is increased when there is an increase in any of the following: peak inspiratory pressure, frequency, inspiratory time. *MAWP* is also increased when expiratory resistance (hold), pressure support, or *PEEP* is applied.

An increase in *MAWP* may cause the cardiac output to fall, particularly in patients with unstable hemodynamic status. An increase in *MAWP* may also cause an increase in intracranial pressure. Therefore, *MAWP* should be kept at the lowest possible level by limiting the factors listed above, particularly the *I* time and *PEEP*.

EQUATION

$$MAWP = \left[\frac{f \times I \text{ time}}{60} \right] \times (PIP - PEEP) + PEEP$$

(Constant pressure ventilation)

$$MAWP = 0.5 \left[\frac{f \times I \text{ time}}{60} \right] \times (PIP - PEEP) + PEEP$$

(Constant flow ventilation)

MAWP	:	Mean airway pressure in cm H_2O ($\bar{P}aw$)
f	:	Frequency/min
I time	:	Inspiratory time in sec
PIP	:	Peak inspiratory pressure in cm H_2O
PEEP	:	Positive end-expiratory pressure in cm H_2O

NORMAL VALUE

Use serial measurements to establish trend.

EXAMPLE 1

When *PEEP* is used:
Given: f = 45/min
      I time = 0.5 sec
      PIP = 35 cm H_2O
      PEEP = 5 cm H_2O
Calculate the mean airway pressure.

$$
\begin{aligned}
MAWP &= \left[\frac{f \times I \text{ time}}{60} \right] \times (PIP - PEEP) + PEEP \\
&= \left[\frac{45 \times 0.5}{60} \right] \times (35 - 5) + 5 \\
&= \left[\frac{22.5}{60} \right] \times 30 + 5 \\
&= [0.375] \times 30 + 5 \\
&= 11.25 + 5 \\
&= 16.25 \text{ or } 16 \text{ cm } H_2O
\end{aligned}
$$

EXAMPLE 2

When *PEEP* is not used (assuming same *PIP*):
Given: f = 45/min
I time   = 0.5 sec
PIP = 35 cm H_2O
$PEEP$ = 0 cm H_2O
Calculate the mean airway pressure.

$$MAWP = \left[\frac{f \times I \text{ time}}{60} \right] \times (PIP - PEEP) + PEEP$$

$$= \left[\frac{45 \times 0.5}{60} \right] \times (35 - 0) + 0$$

$$= \left[\frac{22.5}{60} \right] \times 35 + 0$$

$$= [0.375] \times 35 + 0$$

$$= 13.13 + 0$$

$$= 13.13 \text{ or } 13 \text{ cm } H_2O$$

EXERCISE 1

When *PEEP* is used:
Given: f = 16/min
I time   = 1 sec
PIP = 40 cm H_2O
$PEEP$ = 10 cm H_2O
What is the calculated mean airway pressure?

[Answer: $MAWP$ = 18 cm H_2O]

EXERCISE 2

When *PEEP* is not used (assuming same *PIP*):
Given: f = 16/min
I time   = 1 sec
PIP = 40 cm H_2O
$PEEP$ = 0 cm H_2O
Calculate the mean airway pressure.

[Answer: $MAWP$ = 10.67 or 11 cm H_2O]

REFERENCE

Burton

SELF-ASSESSMENT QUESTIONS

47a. Given: f = 20/min, I time = 0.5 sec, PIP = 40 cm H_2O,
$PEEP$ = 5 cm H_2O. Calculate the mean airway pressure ($MAWP$).

(A) 11 cm H_2O
(B) 13 cm H_2O
(C) 15 cm H_2O
(D) 17 cm H_2O

47b. Given: f = 26/min, I time = 1.0 sec, PIP = 65 cm H_2O,
   $PEEP$ = 15 cm H_2O. Calculate the mean airway pressure (*MAWP*).

   (A) 21.7 cm H_2O
   (B) 30.3 cm H_2O
   (C) 36.7 cm H_2O
   (D) 39.4 cm H_2O

47c. A patient has the following settings on a mechanical ventilator:
   f = 16/min, I time = 1.5 sec, PIP = 50 cm H_2O, $PEEP$ = 0 cm H_2O.
   What is the calculated mean airway pressure (*MAWP*)?

   (A) 16 cm H_2O
   (B) 20 cm H_2O
   (C) 24 cm H_2O
   (D) 30 cm H_2O

47d. Positive end-expiratory pressure (*PEEP*) of 10 cm H_2O is added to
   the patient in the preceding question. The new parameters are as
   follows: f =16/min, I time = 1.5 sec PIP = 55 cm H_2O, $PEEP$ =
   10 cm H_2O. What is the calculated mean airway pressure (*MAWP*)?

   (A) 16 cm H_2O
   (B) 18 cm H_2O
   (C) 23 cm H_2O
   (D) 28 cm H_2O

47e. A neonate is being ventilated by a pressure-limited ventilator with
   these settings: f = 36/min, I time = 0.5 sec, PIP = 35 cm H_2O,
   $PEEP$ = 5 cm H_2O. Based on this information, calculate the
   mean airway pressure (*MAWP*).

   (A) 9 cm H_2O
   (B) 14 cm H_2O
   (C) 20 cm H_2O
   (D) 30 cm H_2O

47f. An infant ventilator has these settings: f = 30/min, I time =
   0.5 sec, PIP = 25 cm H_2O, $PEEP$ = 6 cm H_2O. What is the
   approximate mean airway pressure (*MAWP*)? If the I time is
   increased to 0.6 sec, would the *MAWP* be higher or lower if other
   parameters remain unchanged?

   (A) 9 cm H_2O; higher (10 cm H_2O)
   (B) 11 cm H_2O; lower (10 cm H_2O)
   (C) 11 cm H_2O; higher (12 cm H_2O)
   (D) 17 cm H_2O; higher (18 cm H_2O)

47g. A recent ventilator check in the NICU revealed the following ventilator
   settings: f = 40/min, I time = 0.4 sec, PIP = 30 cm H_2O, $PEEP$ =
   0 cm H_2O. What is the neonate's approximate mean airway pressure
   (*MAWP*)? If *PEEP* of 5 cm H_2O is added to the ventilator settings, what
   will be the new *MAWP* if other parameters remain unchanged?

   (A) 7 cm H_2O; 12 cm H_2O
   (B) 7 cm H_2O; 13 cm H_2O
   (C) 8 cm H_2O; 12 cm H_2O
   (D) 8 cm H_2O; 13 cm H_2O

Chapter

48

Mean Arterial Pressure (*MAP*)

NOTES

This equation calculates the mean (average) arterial blood pressure in the systemic circulation. A normal value of 60 mm Hg is considered the minimum *MAP* needed to maintain adequate tissue perfusion.

MAP is directly related to the systemic vascular resistance (*SVR*) and the cardiac output (*CO*):

$$MAP = SVR \times CO$$

In patients whose systemic vascular resistance is low (e.g., loss of venous tone) or whose cardiac output is low (e.g., CHF), the *MAP* will be low. The *MAP* is usually high in patients with systemic hypertension.

This equation uses $2 \times BP_{\text{diastolic}}$ because the diastolic phase is assumed to be twice as long as the systolic phase. When the heart rate is greater than 120/min, this equation loses its accuracy.

EQUATION

$$MAP = \frac{BP_{\text{systolic}} + 2\ BP_{\text{diastolic}}}{3}$$

MAP : Mean arterial pressure in mm Hg
BP_{systolic} : Systolic blood pressure in mm Hg
$BP_{\text{diastolic}}$: Diastolic blood pressure in mm Hg

NORMAL VALUE >60 mm Hg

EXAMPLE

Given: BP_{systolic} = 120 mm Hg

$BP_{\text{diastolic}}$ = 80 mm Hg

Calculate the mean arterial pressure.

$$MAP = \frac{BP_{\text{systolic}} + 2\ BP_{\text{diastolic}}}{3}$$

$$= \frac{120 + 2 \times 80}{3}$$

$$= \frac{120 + 160}{3}$$

$$= \frac{280}{3}$$

$$= 93 \text{ mm Hg}$$

EXERCISE

Given: Systolic blood pressure = 110 mm Hg

Diastolic blood pressure = 50 mm Hg

Calculate the *MAP*.

[Answer: *MAP* = 70 mm Hg]

REFERENCE Burton

SEE *Vascular Resistance: Systemic (SVR); Cardiac Output (CO): Fick's Estimated Method.*

SELF-ASSESSMENT QUESTIONS

48a. Given: systolic blood pressure = 100 mm Hg, diastolic blood pressure = 60 mm Hg. Calculate the mean arterial pressure (*MAP*).

(A) 60 mm Hg
(B) 73 mm Hg
(C) 80 mm Hg
(D) 100 mm Hg

48b. Given: systolic blood pressure = 110 mm Hg, diastolic blood pressure = 70 mm Hg. Calculate the mean arterial pressure (*MAP*).

(A) 35 mm Hg
(B) 60 mm Hg
(C) 70 mm Hg
(D) 83 mm Hg

48c. A patient has a systemic blood pressure reading of 90/60 mm Hg. The calculated mean arterial pressure (*MAP*) is therefore

(A) 50 mm Hg
(B) 60 mm Hg
(C) 70 mm Hg
(D) 75 mm Hg

48d. The mean arterial pressure is directly related to the:

(A) systemic vascular resistance.
(B) cardiac output.
(C) systolic and diastolic pressures.
(D) All of the above.

Chapter

49

Metric Conversion: Length

If a calculator is used to obtain the answer, the number in front of the decimal point represents the feet; the number after the decimal point should be multiplied by 12 to obtain the remaining height in inches. In Example 4, 63/12 = 5.25, the number in front of the decimal point (5) is the height in feet. The number after the decimal point (0.25) is multiplied by 12 for the remaining height in inches: 0.25 × 12 = 3 inches. The height is therefore 5'3".

In Step 4 of Example 4, the number in front of the decimal point (5) represents the height in ft. The number after the decimal point (0.25) should be multiplied by 12 to convert ft to in (0.25 ft = 0.25 × 12 inches = 3 inches). Therefore, 5.25 ft equals 5 ft 3 in.

CONVERSION TABLE

Millimeters	Centimeters	Inches	Feet	Yards	Meters
1	0.1	0.03937	0.00328	0.00109	0.001
10.0	1	0.3937	0.03281	0.0109	0.01
25.4	2.54	1	0.0833	0.0278	0.0254
304.8	30.48	12.0	1	0.3333	0.3048
914.40	91.44	36.0	3.0	1	0.9144
1000.0	100.0	39.37	3.2808	1.0936	1

EXAMPLE 1

Convert 8 inches (in) to millimeters (mm).
Step 1. From the conversion table, 1 in = 25.4 mm
Step 2. 8 in = (8 × 25.4) mm or 203.2 mm

EXAMPLE 2

Convert 40 centimeters (cm) to feet (ft).
Step 1. From the conversion table, 1 cm = 0.03281 ft
Step 2. 40 cm = (40 × 0.03281) ft or 1.3124 ft

EXAMPLE 3

Mr. James is 5'8" tall. What is the centimeter (cm) equivalent?
Step 1. From the conversion table, 1 ft = 12 in
Step 2. 5 ft = (5 × 12) in = 60 in
Step 3. 5'8" is therefore 68 in (60 + 8)
Step 4. From the conversion table, 1 in = 2.54 cm
Step 5. 68 in = (68 × 2.54) cm or 172.72 cm

EXAMPLE 4

Ms. Malby is 160 cm tall. How tall is she in feet and inches?
Step 1. From the conversion table, 1 cm = 0.3937 in
Step 2. 160 cm = (160 × 0.3937) in = 63 in
Step 3. From the conversion table, 1 ft = 12 in
Step 4. 63 in = (63/12) ft = 5.25 ft or 5'3"

EXERCISE 1

A patient tells you that her height is 5'5". If you need to enter her height in the pulmonary function data sheet in centimeters (cm), what should it be?

[Answer: Height in cm = 165.1 or 165 cm]

EXERCISE 2   Mr. Hall is 176 cm tall. Convert his height to feet and inches.

[Answer: Height in ft and in = 5'9"]

SELF-ASSESSMENT QUESTIONS

49a. Convert 280 millimeters (mm) to inches (in).

 (A) 1.02 in
 (B) 11.02 in
 (C) 110.2 in
 (D) 7112 in

$$\frac{280\,mm}{1} \cdot \frac{0.039\,in}{1\ \ mm} = 10.92$$

49b. Convert 46 meters (m) to feet (ft).

 (A) 14 ft
 (B) 15.1 ft
 (C) 140 ft
 (D) 151 ft

$$\frac{46\,m}{1} \cdot \frac{3.28\,ft}{1\ \ m} = 150.88$$

49c. Convert 12 inches (in) to centimeters (cm).

 (A) 0.30 cm
 (B) 3.05 cm
 (C) 30.48 cm
 (D) 304.8 cm

$$\frac{12\,in}{1} \cdot \frac{2.54\,cm}{1\ \ in} = 30.48$$

49d. Convert 1.6 feet (ft) to millimeters (mm).

 (A) 487.7 mm
 (B) 4,877 mm
 (C) 521.4 mm
 (D) 5,214 mm

$$\frac{1.6\,ft}{1} \cdot \frac{304.8\,mm}{1\ \ ft} = 487.68$$

49e. A patient, Ms. Smith, is 5'6" tall. What is the centimeter (cm) equivalent?

 (A) 154.10 cm
 (B) 1541 cm
 (C) 167.6 cm
 (D) 1,676 cm

$$\frac{5\,ft}{1} \cdot \frac{30.48\,cm}{1\ \ ft} = 152.4\,ft$$

49f. Mr. Jackson is 180 cm tall. Convert this height to feet and inches.

 (A) 5 ft 8 in
 (B) 5 ft 9 in
 (C) 5 ft 10 in
 (D) 5 ft 11 in

$$\frac{180\,cm}{1}\ \frac{0.393\,in}{1\ \ cm} = 70.74\ in$$

$$\frac{70.74\,in\ \ \ \ 0.0833}{1}$$

49g. A patient is 5'9" tall. If you need to record the height in centimeters (cm), what should it be?

(A) 167 cm

(B) 175 cm

(C) 179 cm

(D) 182 cm

49h. Mr. Hall runs 1,600 meters every morning. This is the same as how many feet?

(A) 524 ft

(B) 4,800 ft

(C) 5,249 ft

(D) 48,000 ft

$$1,600 \text{ meters} \cdot \frac{3.28 ft}{1m} = 5,248$$

$$1m = 3.28 ft$$

Chapter

50

Metric Conversion: Volume

CONVERSION TABLE

Milliliters	Microliters	Liters	Fluid Ounces	Pints	Quarts
1	1000	0.001	0.03381	0.00211	0.001055
0.001	1	0.000001	0.0000338	0.00000211	0.000001055
1000	1000000	1	33.8	2.11	1.55
29.57	29570	0.02957	1	0.0625	0.0315
473.16	47316	0.47316	16.0	1	0.5
946.32	94632	0.94632	32.0	2.0	1

EXAMPLE 1

Convert 12 fluid ounces (fl oz) to milliliters (mL).
Step 1. From the conversion table, 1 fl oz = 29.57 mL
Step 2. 12 fl oz = (12 × 29.57) mL or 354.84 mL

EXAMPLE 2

Convert 2 liters (L) to pints (pt).
Step 1. From the conversion table, 1 L = 2.11 pt
Step 2. 2 L = (2 × 2.11) pt or 4.22 pt

EXAMPLE 3

A blood gas analyzer has the capability to analyze blood samples as low as 100 microliters (μL). What is the milliliter (mL) equivalent?
Step 1. From the conversion table, 1 μL = 0.001 mL
Step 2. 100 μL = (100 × 0.001) mL = 0.1 mL

EXAMPLE 4

A large-volume aerosol unit holds 1,000 ml of sterile water. Convert this volume to fluid ounces (fl oz).
Step 1. From the conversion table, 1 mL = 0.03381 fl oz
Step 2. 1,000 mL = (1,000 × 0.03381) fl oz = 33.81 fl oz

EXERCISE 1

In order to analyze a capillary blood gas sample, a minimum sample size of 60 microliters (μL) is needed. What is the milliliter (mL) equivalent?

[Answer: Sample size in mL = 0.06 mL]

EXERCISE 2

Before using a concentrated disinfectant solution, 2 liters of water must be added. How much water in fluid ounces (fl oz) should be added to prepare this disinfectant solution before use?

[Answer: Water to be added = 67.6 fl oz]

SELF-ASSESSMENT QUESTIONS

50a. Convert 32 fluid ounces (fl oz) to milliliters (mL).

(A) 1.08 mL
(B) 94.6 mL
(C) 946 mL
(D) 1,008 mL

50b. Convert 6 pints (pt) to liters.

(A) 2.12 L
(B) 2.84 L
(C) 21.2 L
(D) 28.4 L

50c. Convert 2 liters (L) to milliliters (mL).

(A) 20 mL
(B) 200 mL
(C) 2,000 mL
(D) 20,000 mL

50d. Convert 300 microliters (μL) to milliliters (mL).

(A) 0.003 mL
(B) 0.03 mL
(C) 0.3 mL
(D) 3 mL

50e. A blood gas syringe contains 0.4 mL of arterial blood sample. What is the microliters (μL) equivalent?

(A) 0.4 μL
(B) 4 μL
(C) 40 μL
(D) 400 μL

50f. A heated cascade holds 1.6 quarts of sterile water. Convert this volume to liters (L).

(A) 1.51 L
(B) 1.78 L
(C) 15.1 L
(D) 17.8 L

50g. The minimum sample size for a blood gas analyzer is 80
     microliters (μL). What is the milliliter (mL) equivalent?

(A) 0.008 mL
(B) 0.08 mL
(C) 0.8 mL
(D) 8 mL

50h. A concentrated cleaning solution is being diluted with 12 quarts
     of water before use. How much water in fluid ounces (fl oz)
     should be added?

(A) 36.5 fl oz
(B) 365 fl oz
(C) 38.4 fl oz
(D) 384 fl oz

Chapter

51

Metric Conversion: Weight

NOTES

In step 2 of example 4, the number in front of the decimal point represents the weight in lb. The number after the decimal point should be multiplied by 16 to obtain the remaining weight in oz. In this example, 1 (the number in front of the decimal point) is the weight in lb; 0.76 (the number after the decimal point) is multiplied by 16 for the remaining weight in oz: 0.76 × 16 = 12.16 oz or 12 oz. The birth weight is therefore 1 lb 12 oz.

CONVERSION TABLE

Milligrams	Grams	Kilograms	Ounces	Pounds
1	0.001	0.000001	0.0000352	0.0000022
1000	1	0.001	0.0352	0.0022
1000000	1000	1	35.2	2.2
28410	28.41	0.02841	1	0.0625
454545	454.545	0.4545	16.0	1

EXAMPLE 1

Convert 78 kilograms (kg) to pounds (lb).
Step 1. From the conversion table, 1 kg = 2.2 lb
Step 2. 78 kg = (78 × 2.2) lb or 171.6 lb

EXAMPLE 2

Convert 120 pounds (lb) to kilograms (kg).
Step 1. From the conversion table, 1 lb = 0.4545 kg
Step 2. 120 lb = (120 × 0.4545) or 54.54 kg

EXAMPLE 3

Convert 6 lb 7 oz to grams (gm) and kilograms (kg).
Step 1. From the conversion table, 1 lb = 16 oz
Step 2. 6 lb = (6 × 16) oz = 96 oz
Step 3. 6 lb 7 oz = (96 + 7) oz = 103 oz
Step 4. From the conversion table, 1 oz = 28.41 gm
Step 5. 103 oz = (103 × 28.41) gm = 2,926.23 gm
Step 6. From the conversion table, 1 gm = 0.001 kg
Step 7. 2,926.23 gm = (2,926.23 × 0.001) = 2.92623 or 2.93 kg
6 lb 7 oz = 2,926.23 gm or 2.93 kg

EXAMPLE 4

A premature infant weights 800 grams (g) at birth. What is this birth weight in pounds (lb) and ounces (oz)?
Step 1. From the conversion table, 1 g = 0.0022 lb
Step 2. 800 g = (800 × 0.0022) lb = 1.76 lb or 1 lb 12 oz
800 gm = 1 lb 12 oz

EXERCISE 1   Mr. Dade, who weighs 150 lbs, is ready for the pulmonary function study. What is his weight in kilograms (kg)?

[Answer: Weight = 68.18 kg]

EXERCISE 2   The birth weight of a neonate is 3 lb 12 oz. What is this birth weight in grams (gm) and kilograms (kg)?

[Answer: Birth weight = 1,704.6 gm or 1.7 kg]

SELF-ASSESSMENT QUESTIONS

51a. Convert 1,200 grams (g) to pounds (lb).

(A) 0.26 lb
(B) 0.32 lb
(C) 2.64 lb
(D) 3.18 lb

51b. Convert 150 pounds (lb) to kilograms (kg).

(A) 59.22 kg
(B) 62.15 kg
(C) 68.18 kg
(D) 70.02 kg

51c. Convert 77 kilograms (kg) to pounds (lb).

(A) 169.4 lb
(B) 172.9 lb
(C) 174.2 lb
(D) 177.7 lb

51d. Convert 8 lb 4 oz to grams (gm).

(A) 3,675 gm
(B) 3,700 gm
(C) 3,725 gm
(D) 3,750 gm

51e. Convert 8 lb 7 oz to kilograms (kg).

(A) 3.66 kg
(B) 3.84 kg
(C) 4.07 kg
(D) 4.22 kg

51f. A neonate weighs 3,500 grams (g) at birth. Record this birth weight in pounds (lb) and ounces (oz).

(A) 7 lb 7 oz
(B) 7 lb 11 oz
(C) 7 lb 14 oz
(D) 8 lb 1 oz

51g. The birth weight of a neonate is 4 lb 6 oz. What is this birth weight in grams (gm) and kilograms (kg)?

(A) 181.8 gm, 18.18 kg
(B) 1,818 gm, 1.82 kg
(C) 198.8 gm, 1.99 kg
(D) 1,988 gm, 1.99 kg

51h. A concentration of 1 g per 100 mL is the same as _____ mg per 100 mL.

(A) 10
(B) 100
(C) 1,000
(D) 10,000

51i. An 0.5% bronchodilator solution has a concentration of 0.5 g per 100 mL. This is the same as how many milligrams per 100 mL?

(A) 500 mg
(B) 5,000 mg
(C) 50,000 mg
(D) 500,000 mg

Chapter

52

Minute Ventilation During IMV

EQUATION

$$\dot{V}_E = (V_T \text{ mech} \times f \text{ mech}) + (V_T \text{ spon} \times f \text{ spon})$$

$\dot{V}_E$	:	Expired minute ventilation in L/min
V_T mech	:	Mechanical ventilator tidal volume in mL
f mech	:	Mechanical ventilator frequency/min
V_T spon	:	Patient's spontaneous tidal volume in mL
f spon	:	Patient's spontaneous frequency/min

EXAMPLE

Given: V_T mech $= 700$ mL
$\quad\quad\quad f$ mech $= 8$/min
$\quad\quad\quad V_T$ spon $= 250$ mL
$\quad\quad\quad f$ spon $= 10$/min
Calculate the expired minute ventilation ($\dot{V}_E$).
$\dot{V}_E = (V_T \text{ mech} \times f \text{ mech}) + (V_T \text{ spon} \times f \text{ spon})$
$\quad\quad = (700 \times 8) + (250 \times 10)$
$\quad\quad = 5,600 + 2,500$
$\quad\quad = 8,100$ mL/min or 8.1 L/min

EXERCISE

Given: V_T mech $= 600$ mL
$\quad\quad\quad f$ mech $= 10$/min
$\quad\quad\quad V_T$ spon $= 240$ mL
$\quad\quad\quad f$ spon $= 10$/min
Calculate the expired minute ventilation ($\dot{V}_E$).

[Answer: $\dot{V}_E = 8.4$ L/min]

SEE

Corrected Tidal Volume (V_T).

SELF-ASSESSMENT QUESTIONS

52a. Given: V_T mech $= 500$ mL, f mech $= 10$/min, V_T spon $= 200$ mL, f spon $= 10$/min. Calculate the approximate minute ventilation ($\dot{V}_E$).

(A) 4 L
(B) 5 L
(C) 6 L
(D) 7 L

[handwritten:] $\dot{V}_E = (500 \times 10) + (200 \times 10)$
$5,000 + 2,000$
$= 7,000 \text{ mL} \rightarrow 7\text{L}$

52b. The following average measurements are obtained from a ventilator check while the patient is on the SIMV mode: V_T mech = 600 mL, f mech = 12/min, V_T spon = 260 mL, f spon = 10/min. What is the minute ventilation?

(A) 3.5 L
(B) 7.2 L
(C) 9.8 L
(D) 10.7 L

$$(600 \times 12) + (260 \times 10)$$
$$7,200 + 2,600$$
$$9,800 \text{ mL} \rightarrow 9.8 \text{ L}$$

52c. While on the SIMV mode, a patient was breathing spontaneously at a rate of 6/min and an average tidal volume of 300 mL. If the ventilator tidal volume and rate were set at 650 mL and 10/min, respectively, what is the approximate minute ventilation?

(A) 7.5 L
(B) 8.3 L
(C) 9.4 L
(D) 10.8 L

$$(300 \times 6) + (650 \times 10)$$
$$1,800 + 6,500$$
$$8,300 \text{ mL} \rightarrow 8.3 \text{ L}$$

Chapter

53

Minute Ventilation: Expired and Alveolar

NOTES

These equations are used to calculate the expired minute ventilation and the alveolar minute ventilation.

The expired minute ventilation ($\dot{V}_E$) estimates a patient's ventilation effort (Figure 2-32). The alveolar minute ventilation ($\dot{V}_A$) is more meaningful; it accurately reflects the effective ventilation—the portion of ventilation capable of taking part in gas exchange (Figure 2-33).

Normally 1 mL/lb body weight is used to estimate the anatomic deadspace. If the physiologic deadspace is significant, the V_D should be measured.

In mechanical ventilation, the V_T should be the corrected tidal volume.

EQUATION 1

$$\dot{V}_E = V_T \times f$$

EQUATION 2

$$\dot{V}_A = (V_T - V_D) \times f$$

$\dot{V}_E$: Expired minute ventilation in L/min

$\dot{V}_A$: Alveolar minute ventilation in L/min

V_T : Tidal volume in mL

V_D : Deadspace volume in mL

f : Respiratory frequency/min

EXAMPLE

Given: $V_T = 600$ mL
$V_D = 150$ mL
$f = 12$/min

Calculate the expired minute ventilation ($\dot{V}_E$) and the alveolar minute ventilation ($\dot{V}_A$).

$$\dot{V}_E = V_T \times f$$
$$= 600 \times 12$$
$$= 7{,}200 \text{ mL/min or } 7.2 \text{ L/min}$$
$$\dot{V}_A = (V_T - V_D) \times f$$
$$= (600 - 150) \times 12$$
$$= 450 \times 12$$
$$= 5{,}400 \text{ mL/min or } 5.4 \text{ L/min}$$

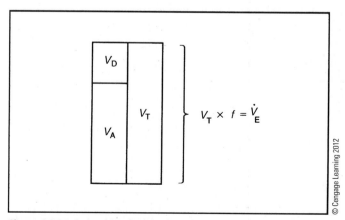

Figure 2-32 Relationship of tidal volume (V_T) and expired minute ventilation ($\dot{V}_E$). f is respiratory frequency per minute.

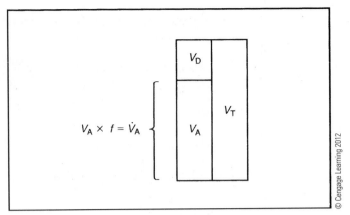

Figure 2-33 Relationship of alveolar volume (V_A) and alveolar minute ventilation ($\dot{V}_A$). f is respiratory frequency per minute.

EXERCISE	Given: V_T = 550 mL
	V_D = 100 mL
	f = 12/min

Calculate the $\dot{V}_E$ and the $\dot{V}_A$.

[Answer: $\dot{V}_E$ = 6.6 L/min $\dot{V}_A$ = 5.4 L/min]

REFERENCE   Madama

SEE   *Deadspace to Tidal Volume Ratio (V_D/V_T);*

Corrected Tidal Volume (V_T).

SELF-ASSESSMENT QUESTIONS

53a. The anatomic deadspace can be estimated to be:

(A) 1 mL/kg of body weight.
(B) 1 mL/lb of body weight.
(C) 10 mL/kg of body weight.
(D) 10 mL/lb of body weight.

53b. A patient has an expired tidal volume of 600 mL. If the patient weights 120 lb, the estimated alveolar tidal volume is:

(A) 600 mL.
(B) 520 mL.
(C) 480 mL.
(D) 420 mL.

53c. A patient has a tidal volume of 600 mL and a respiratory frequency of 12/min. What is the patient's expired minute ventilation?

(A) 3.8 L
(B) 4.4 L
(C) 5.4 L
(D) 7.2 L

For questions 53d-53f: V_T = 800 mL, V_D = 200 mL, f = 10/min.

53d. What is the alveolar minute ventilation?

(A) 600 mL
(B) 800 mL
(C) 6 L
(D) 8 L

53e. What is the alveolar tidal volume?

(A) 200 mL
(B) 400 mL
(C) 600 mL
(D) 800 mL

53f. The calculated $\dot{V}_E$ is:

(A) 600 mL.
(B) 800 mL.
(C) 6 L.
(D) 8 L.

53g. A patient is breathing at a tidal volume of 600 mL and a frequency of 12/min. What is the estimated alveolar minute ventilation if the patient weighs 150 lb?

(A) 3.8 L
(B) 4.4 L
(C) 5.4 L
(D) 6.8 L

53h. Exhaled volumes are collected from a patient over a 1-min interval; during this time 14 breaths are recorded. If the total expired volume is 10 L, the average tidal volume is about:

(A) 140 mL.
(B) 714 mL.
(C) 1,000 mL.
(D) 1,100 mL.

53i. What is the expected alveolar minute ventilation for a 68 kg (150 lb) patient who has a tidal volume of 500 mL and a frequency of 20/min?

(A) 3 L
(B) 7 L
(C) 8 L
(D) 9 L

53j. Given: $V_T = 780$ mL, $V_D = 160$ mL, $f = 14$/min. Calculate the approximate expired minute ventilation ($\dot{V}_E$) and alveolar minute ventilation ($\dot{V}_A$).

(A) 7.8 L; 6.2 L
(B) 9.4 L; 7.8 L
(C) 10.9 L; 7.8 L
(D) 10.9 L; 8.7 L

53k. A patient weighing 130 lb has an average V_T of 610 mL and frequency of 16/min. What is the estimated deadspace volume (V_D)? What is the calculated alveolar minute ventilation ($\dot{V}_A$)?

(A) 100 mL; 6.10 L
(B) 100 mL; 7.68 L
(C) 130 mL; 7.68 L
(D) 130 mL; 9.76 L

53l. Which of the following measurements provide the largest alveolar minute ventilation?

	V_T (mL)	V_D (mL)	f
(A)	800	110	15
(B)	750	130	18
(C)	760	140	14
(D)	690	120	16

53m. Based on the equation $\dot{V}_A = (V_T - V_D) \times f$, the alveolar minute ventilation ($\dot{V}_A$) may be increased by all of the following *except*:

(A) increasing the V_T.
(B) decreasing the V_T.
(C) decreasing the V_D.
(D) increasing the f.

54

Oxygen:Air (O_2:Air) Entrainment Ratio

This equation calculates the O_2:air entrainment ratio at any F_IO_2 between 21% and 99%.

In the equation shown, the 21 represents the oxygen fraction of room air. The 21 should not be rounded off to 20 in calculations involving F_IO_2 of less than 30% because rounding off can cause erroneous results.

To find the total flow of a venturi device, simply add the O_2:air ratio and then multiply the sum by the oxygen flow rate. For example, the O_2:air ratio for 28% oxygen is 1:10 so therefore, the total flow of a 28% oxygen venturi device running at 4 L/min of oxygen is $(1 + 10) \times 4$ or 44 L/min.

EQUATION

$$O_2\text{:air} = 1 : \frac{100 - F_IO_2}{F_IO_2 - 21}$$

O_2:air : Oxygen:air entrainment ratio

F_IO_2 : Inspired oxygen concentration in %

EXAMPLE 1

Find the O_2:air ratio of 28% oxygen.

$$O_2\text{:air} = 1 : \frac{100 - 28}{28 - 21}$$

$$= 1 : \frac{72}{7}$$

$$= 1 : 10.3 \text{ or } 1:10$$

At 28% oxygen, every 1 unit of oxygen is mixed with 10 units of air. See Figure 2-34 for the progression of a "tick-tack-toe" method to solve this problem.

21 — 100 — F_IO_2 — — — —	21 — 100 — 28 — — — —	21 — 100 — 28 — 72 / −7 = 10.3
Set up tick-tack-toe as above.	To find O_2: air ratio for 28% oxygen, write 28% in the F_IO_2 block.	Subtract the numbers diagonally. Divide the resulting numbers (72/7). The ratio is 1:10.3 or 1:10. [Disregard the minus sign]

© Cengage Learning 2012

Figure 2-34 A "tick-tack-toe" method to solve for O_2: air entrainment ratio of 28% oxygen. The number 21 represents the percentage of oxygen in room air, and 100 represents the percentage of oxygen from a pure oxygen source.

EXAMPLE 2   Find the O_2:air ratio of 70% oxygen.

$$O_2\text{:air} = 1 : \frac{100 - 70}{70 - 21}$$

$$= 1 : \frac{30}{49}$$

$$= 1 : 0.61 \text{ or } 1 : 0.6$$

At 70% oxygen, every 1 unit of oxygen is mixed with 0.6 units of air. See Figure 2-35 for the progession of another "tick-tack-toe" method to solve this problem.

21 — 100 — F_IO_2 — — — —	21 — 100 — 70 — — — —	21 — 100 — 70 — 30 / — 49 = 0.61
Set up tick-tack-toe as above.	To find O_2: air ratio for 70% oxygen, write 70% in the F_IO_2 block.	Subtract the numbers diagonally. Divide the resulting numbers (30/49). The ratio is 1:0.61 or 1:0.6. [Disregard the minus sign]

© Cengage Learning 2012

Figure 2-35 A "tick-tack-toe" method to solve for O_2:air entrainment ratio of 28% oxygen. The number 21 represents the percentage of oxygen in room air, and 100 represents the percentage of oxygen from a pure oxygen source.

EXERCISE 1   Find the O_2:air ratio of a 24% oxygen venturi device.

[Answer: O_2:air = 1 : 25.33 or 1 : 25]

EXERCISE 2   What is the total flow of this 24% oxygen venturi device if an oxygen flow rate of 4 L/min is used?

[Answer: Total flow rate = 104 L/min]

REFERENCES   Barnes; White

SELF-ASSESSMENT QUESTIONS

54a. The oxygen:air entrainment ratio for 60% oxygen is:

(A) 1 : 0.7.
(B) 1 : 1.
(C) 1 : 3.
(D) 1 : 5.

54b. Calculate the O_2:air ratio of 30% oxygen.

(A) 1 : 7.8
(B) 1 : 8.1
(C) 1 : 8.9
(D) 1 : 10

54c. An oxygen flow rate of 12 L/min is used on a 60% venturi mask. What is the O_2:air entrainment ratio of the venturi mask? What is the total flow at this oxygen flow rate?

(A) 1 : 0.6; 19.2 L/min

(B) 1 : 1; 24 L/min

(C) 1 : 1; 26.4 L/min

(D) 1 : 1.6; 31.2 L/min

54d. What is the total flow of a 40% venturi mask running at 6 L/min of oxygen?

(A) 12.6 L/min

(B) 18.2 L/min

(C) 24.9 L/min

(D) 28.5 L/min

54e. If a patient is using a 40% venturi mask and a total flow of 36 L/min is desired, what should be the minimum oxygen flow rate?

(A) 6 L/min

(B) 7 L/min

(C) 8 L/min

(D) 9 L/min

54f. A venturi aerosol unit is used to deliver 50% oxygen with aerosol to a patient. What is the oxygen:air ratio at this F_1O_2? What is the total flow at 6 L/min of oxygen?

(A) 1 : 1.5; 13.8 L/min

(B) 1 : 1.5; 15 L/min

(C) 1 : 1.7; 16.2 L/min

(D) 1 : 1.7; 17.4 L/min

54g. A patient is receiving 35% oxygen via a venturi mask at 6 L/min of oxygen. What is the total flow available to this patient? If the patient's minute ventilation is 11 L/min, would the total flow of this venturi setup satisfy the patient's ventilation needs?

(A) 12.8 L/min; no

(B) 27.6 L/min; yes

(C) 27.6 L/min; no

(D) 33.8 L/min; yes

Chapter

55

Oxygen Consumption ($\dot{V}O_2$) and Index ($\dot{V}O_2$ Index)

NOTES

As shown in the example, a person who has a cardiac output ($\dot{Q}_T$) of 5 L/min and an arterial mixed venous oxygen content difference $[C(a - \bar{v})O_2]$ of 4 vol% consumes 200 mL of oxygen per minute. Under normal conditions, oxygen consumption ($\dot{V}O_2$) is directly related to $\dot{Q}_T$ and $[C(a - \bar{v})O_2]$.

Conditions leading to higher oxygen consumption (e.g., exercise) cause the cardiac output ($\dot{Q}_T$) to increase. If the cardiac output fails to keep up with the oxygen consumption needs, the $C(a - \bar{v})O_2$ increases. Some factors that increase oxygen consumption are listed in Table 2-5.

On the other hand, conditions leading to lower oxygen consumption (e.g., skeletal relaxation) cause the cardiac output to decrease. If the cardiac output provides an oxygen level higher than that required or consumed by the body, the $C(a - \bar{v})O_2$ decreases. Some factors that decrease oxygen consumption are listed in Table 2-6.

The oxygen consumption index ($\dot{V}O_2$ index) is used to normalize oxygen consumption measurements among patients of varying body size. The example shows that a $\dot{V}O_2$ index of 143 mL/min/m^2 is normal for an average-sized person ($BSA = 1.4$ m^2) but low ($\dot{V}O_2$ index = 100 mL/min/m^2) for a large person ($BSA = 2$ m^2).

EQUATION 1

$$\dot{V}O_2 = Q_T \times C(a - \bar{v})O_2$$

EQUATION 2

$$\dot{V}O_2 \text{ Index} = \frac{\dot{V}O_2}{BSA}$$

$\dot{V}O_2$: Oxygen consumption in mL/min; oxygen uptake

$\dot{V}O_2$ index : Oxygen consumption index in L/min/m^2

$\dot{Q}_T$: Cardiac output in L/min; CO

$C(a - \bar{v})O_2$: Arterial-mixed venous oxygen content difference in vol%

BSA : Body surface area in m^2

NORMAL VALUES

$\dot{V}O_2$ = 200 to 350 mL/min
$\dot{V}O_2$ index = 125 to 165 mL/min/m^2

EXAMPLE

Given: $\dot{Q}_T$ = 5 L/min
$C(a - \bar{v})O_2$ = 4 vol%
BSA = 1.4m^2 (patient 1) and
BSA = 2 m^2 (patient 2)

Calculate the oxygen consumption and oxygen consumption indices for both patients.

$$\dot{V}O_2 = \dot{Q}_T \times C(a - \bar{v})O_2$$

$$= 5 \text{ L/min} \times 4 \text{ vol\%}$$
$$= 5 \text{ L/min} \times 0.04$$
$$= 0.2 \text{ L/min}$$
$$= 200 \text{ mL/min}$$

$$\dot{V}O_2 \text{ index for patient 1} = \frac{\dot{V}O_2}{BSA \text{ of patient 1}}$$

$$= \frac{200}{1.4}$$

$$= 143 \text{ mL/min/m}^2$$

$$\dot{V}O_2 \text{ index for patient 2} = \frac{\dot{V}O_2}{BSA \text{ of patient 2}}$$

$$= \frac{200}{2}$$

$$= 100 \text{ mL/min/m}^2$$

TABLE 2-5. Factors That Increase Oxygen Consumption

Exercise

Seizures

Shivering in postoperative patient

Hyperthermia

EXERCISE

Given: $\dot{Q}_T = 4.5$ L/min

$C(a - \bar{v})O_2 = 5$ vol%
$BSA = 1.2\ m^2$
Calculate the oxygen consumption and oxygen consumption indices. Are they within normal limits?

[Answer: $\dot{V}O_2 = 225$ mL/min; normal. $\dot{V}O_2$ index = 187.5 mL/min/m^2; abnormal]

TABLE 2-6. Factors That Decrease Oxygen Consumption

Skeletal relaxation (e.g., induced by drugs)

Peripheral shunting (e.g., sepsis, trauma)

Certain poisons (e.g., cyanide prevents cellular metabolism)

Hypothermia

REFERENCES   Des Jardins; Kacmarek

SEE   *Arterial–Mixed Venous Oxygen Content Difference [C(a − v̄)O₂]; Cardiac Output (CO): Fick's Estimated Method; Appendix I, DuBois Body Surface Chart.*

SELF-ASSESSMENT QUESTIONS

55a. Oxygen consumption ($\dot{V}O_2$) in mL/min, is calculated by:

  (A) $\dot{Q}_T \times C(a - v)O_2$

  (B) $\dfrac{\dot{Q}_T}{C(a - v)O_2}$

  (C) $\dot{Q}_T + C(a - v)O_2$

  (D) $\dot{Q}_T - C(a - v)O_2$

55b. The normal oxygen consumption ($\dot{V}O_2$) rate for an adult is between:

  (A) 80 and 120 mL/min.

  (B) 120 and 200 mL/min.

  (C) 200 and 350 mL/min.

  (D) 350 and 500 mL/min.

$\dot{V}O_2 = Q_T \times C(a-\bar{v})O_2$

55c. Given: cardiac output $\dot{Q}_T$ = 5.0 L/min, arterial–mixed venous oxygen content difference $[C(a-\bar{v})O_2]$ = 3.5 vol%, body surface area (*BSA*) = 1.6 m². Calculate the oxygen consumption ($\dot{V}O_2$) rate.

(A) 130 mL/min   *5.0 L/min ∘ 3.5 vol %*

(B) 145 mL/min

(C) 160 mL/min   *∘ 0.35 vol %*

(D) 175 mL/min   *0.175 L = 175 mL/min*

55d. A patient whose body surface area is 1.4 m² has a measured oxygen consumption ($\dot{V}O_2$) of 200 mL/min. What is the calculated oxygen consumption index ($\dot{V}O_2$ index)?

(A) 117 mL/min/m² $\dfrac{VO_2}{BSA} = \dfrac{200 \text{ mL/min}}{1.4 \text{ m}^2}$

(B) 120 mL/min/m²

(C) 130 mL/min/m²

(D) 143 mL/min/m²

55e. Given: cardiac output $\dot{Q}_T$ = 3.6 L/min, arterial–mixed venous oxygen content difference $[C(a-\bar{v})O_2]$ = 4.0 vol%, body surface area (*BSA*) = 1.0 m². Calculate the oxygen consumption ($\dot{V}O_2$) and its index ($\dot{V}O_2$ index).

(A) 132 mL/min; 144 mL/min/m²   *3.6 L/min ∘ .04 = 0.144 L →*

(B) 144 mL/min; 144 mL/min/m²   *144 mL*

(C) 150 mL/min; 150 mL/min/m² $\dfrac{144}{1.0 \text{ m}^2}$ *= 144 (VO₂ index) ↑*

(D) 165 mL/min; 150 mL/min/m²   *(VO₂)*

55f. Which of the following measurements has the highest oxygen consumption rate?

	Q_T (L/min)	$C(a-\bar{v})O_2$ (vol%)	
(A)	5.5	3.9	*= 21.45*
(B)	3.9	4.9	*= 19.11*
(C)	3.2	5.0	*= 16*
(D)	4.7	4.1	*= 19.27*

55g. Which of the following measurements has the highest oxygen consumption index?

	Q_T (L/min)	$C(a-\bar{v})O_2$ (vol%)	Body surface area (m²)	
(A)	3.4	5.3 *= 18.02*	1.6	*= 11.26*
(B)	3.9	4.9 *= 19.11*	1.5	*= 12.74*
(C)	4.2	5.0 *= 21.00*	1.7	*= 12.35*
(D)	4.7	4.1 *= 19.27*	1.9	*= 10.14*

Chapter

56

Oxygen Content: Arterial (C_aO_2)

NOTES

C_aO_2 reflects the overall oxygen-carrying capacity of arterial blood. The major determinants of oxygen content are the hemoglobin (Hb) level and the oxygen saturation (S_aO_2). In normal arterial blood gases, the amount of dissolved O_2 contributes only about 0.3 vol% to the oxygen content of 20 vol% (Figure 2-36).

A low Hb level (e.g., anemia) or a low O_2 saturation (e.g., hypoxia) significantly lowers the arterial oxygen content. On the other hand, a high Hb level (e.g., polycythemia) or high O_2 saturation (e.g., hyperoxia) raises the arterial oxygen content.

EQUATION

$$C_aO_2 = (Hb \times 1.34 \times S_aO_2) + (P_aO_2 \times 0.003)$$

C_aO_2	:	Arterial oxygen content in vol%
Hb	:	Hemoglobin content in g%
1.34	:	Amount of oxygen that 1 g of fully saturated hemoglobin can hold
S_aO_2	:	Arterial oxygen saturation in %
P_aO_2	:	Arterial oxygen tension in mm Hg
0.003	:	Amount of dissolved oxygen for 1 mm Hg of P_aO_2

NORMAL VALUE

16 to 20 vol%

EXAMPLE

Given: Hb $=$ 15 g%
$S_aO_2 =$ 98%
$P_aO_2 =$ 100 mm Hg
Calculate the arterial oxygen content.

$$
\begin{aligned}
C_aO_2 &= (Hb \times 1.34 \times S_aO_2) + (P_aO_2 \times 0.003) \\
&= (15 \times 1.34 \times 98\%) + (100 \times 0.003) \\
&= 19.70 + 0.3 \\
&= 20 \text{ vol\%}
\end{aligned}
$$

EXERCISE

Given: Hb $=$ 10 g%
$S_aO_2 =$ 80%
$P_aO_2 =$ 60 mm Hg
Calculate the C_aO_2.

[Answer: C_aO_2 = 10.9 vol%]

REFERENCES

Burton; Shapiro

SEE

Oxygen Content: Mixed Venous ($C_{\bar{v}}O_2$); Oxygen Content: End-capillary (C_cO_2).

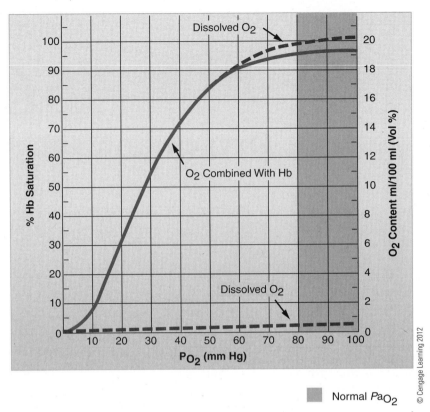

Figure 2-36 Oxygen dissociation curve

SELF-ASSESSMENT QUESTIONS

56a. When the P_aO_2 is 50 mm Hg, the amount of oxygen dissolved in 100 mL of blood is about:

   (A) 0.05 mL.
   (B) 0.10 mL.
   (C) 0.15 mL.
   (D) 0.20 mL.

56b. The amount of oxygen bound to the hemoglobin (Hb) is normally calculated by using the equation:

   (A) $Hb \times 1.34 + P_aO_2 \times 0.003$
   (B) $Hb \times 1.34$
   (C) $Hb \times 1.34 \times S_aO_2$
   (D) $Hb \times S_aO_2$

56c. In 100 mL of blood, 1 g of hemoglobin when fully saturated with oxygen can carry:

   (A) 100 mL oxygen.
   (B) 40 mL oxygen.
   (C) 47 mL oxygen.
   (D) 1.34 mL oxygen.

56d. The sum of the oxygen attached to hemoglobin and that dissolved in plasma is called:

(A) oxygen content.

(B) oxygen tension.

(C) oxygen concentration.

(D) oxygen saturation.

56e. What is the arterial oxygen content of an individual who has a P_aO_2 of 300 mm Hg, oxygen saturation of 99%, and hemoglobin of 16 g?

(A) 22.1 mL

(B) 21.7 mL

(C) 21.4 mL

(D) 19.6 mL

56f. Given: Hb = 10 g%, S_aO_2 = 95%, P_aO_2 = 60 mm Hg. The calculated C_aO_2 is:

(A) 11.1 vol%.

(B) 12.9 vol%.

(C) 15.6 vol%.

(D) 17.3 vol%.

56g. Given: Hb = 15 g. What is the estimated C_aO_2 under normal conditions?

(A) 19 vol%

(B) 20 vol%

(C) 21 vol%

(D) 22 vol%

56h. What is the arterial oxygen content (C_aO_2) of a patient who has a P_aO_2 of 100 mm Hg, oxygen saturation of 98%, and a hemoglobin of 12 g/100 mL of blood?

(A) 14 vol%

(B) 15 vol%

(C) 16 vol%

(D) 17 vol%

56i. Given: Hb = 10 g%, S_aO_2 = 90%, P_aO_2 = 80 mm Hg. Calculate the arterial oxygen content (C_aO_2).

(A) 10.2 vol%

(B) 11.1 vol%

(C) 12.3 vol%

(D) 13.4 vol%

56j. A polycythemic patient has the following blood gas values: Hb = 17 g%, S_aO_2 = 90%, P_aO_2 = 60 mm Hg. Based on these results, what is the calculated arterial oxygen content (C_aO_2)?

(A) 19.4 vol%

(B) 19.6 vol%

(C) 20.5 vol%

(D) 20.7 vol%

56k. Which of the following blood gas measurements has the lowest calculated arterial oxygen content (C_aO_2)?

	Hb (g%)	S_aO_2 (%)	P_aO_2 (mm Hg)
(A)	13	98	100
(B)	15	70	55
(C)	16	80	76
(D)	14	85	82

56l. The blood gas measurements of a patient recovering from massive blood loss are as follows: Hb = 8 g%, S_aO_2 = 98%, P_aO_2 = 100 mm Hg. What is the calculated C_aO_2? Is it normal?

(A) 10.1 vol%; normal

(B) 10.1 vol%; abnormal

(C) 10.5 vol%; normal

(D) 10.8 vol%; abnormal

57

Oxygen Content: End-Capillary (C_cO_2)

NOTES

C_cO_2 is a calculated value representing the best oxygen content possible at the pulmonary end-capillary level. It is used in other calculations such as the shunt equation.

End-capillary oxygen content reflects the optimal oxygen-carrying capacity of the cardiopulmonary system. The oxygen saturation is assumed to be 100%. The major determinant of C_cO_2 is the hemoglobin (Hb) level. A low Hb level (e.g., anemia) significantly lowers the end-capillary oxygen content.

EQUATION

$C_cO_2 = (\text{Hb} \times 1.34 \times S_aO_2) + (P_AO_2 \times 0.003)$*

C_cO_2 : End-capillary oxygen content in vol%

Hb : Hemoglobin content in g%

1.34 : Amount of oxygen that 1 g of fully saturated hemoglobin can hold

S_aO_2 : Arterial oxygen saturation, assumed to be 100% in C_cO_2 calculations

P_AO_2 : Alveolar oxygen tension in mm Hg, used in place of end-capillary PO_2 (P_cO_2)

0.003 : Amount of dissolved oxygen for 1 mm Hg of P_aO_2

NORMAL VALUE

Varies according to the hemoglobin level and the F_IO_2.

EXAMPLE

Given: Hb = 15 g%

$\quad\quad\quad F_IO_2$ = 21% [$P_AO_2 = 100$ mm Hg]

Calculate the end-capillary oxygen content (C_cO_2).

$C_cO_2 = (\text{Hb} \times 1.34 \times S_aO_2) + (P_AO_2 \times 0.003)$

$\quad\quad = (15 \times 1.34 \times 100\%) + (100 \times 0.003)$

$\quad\quad = 20.1 + 0.3$

$\quad\quad = 20.4$ vol%

EXERCISE

Given: Hb = 10 g%

$\quad\quad\quad F_IO_2$ = 40% [From Appendix B: $P_AO_2 = 235$ mm Hg]

Calculate the C_cO_2.

[Answer: $C_cO_2 = 14.11$ vol%]

REFERENCES

Burton; Shapiro

SEE

Oxygen Content: Arterial (C_aO_2); Oxygen Content: Mixed Venous ($C_{\bar{v}}O_2$); Appendix X: P_AO_2 at selected F_IO_2.

SELF-ASSESSMENT QUESTIONS

57a. Which of the following calculations requires a P_AO_2 value?

(A) $C_{\bar{v}}O_2$
(B) C_aO_2
(C) C_cO_2
(D) $\dfrac{V_D}{V_T}$

57b. Given: Hb = 14 g%, F_IO_2 = 21% (P_AO_2 = 100 mm Hg).
Calculate the end-capillary oxygen content (C_cO_2).

(A) 18.8 vol%
(B) 19.1 vol%
(C) 20.1 vol%
(D) 21 vol%

Handwritten: $Hb \times 1.34 \times SaO_2 + (PaO_2 \times .003)$

Handwritten: $14 \times 1.34 \times$ ~~X~~ 100%
18.76 + 0.3 = 19.06%

57c. Given: Hb = 15 g%; F_IO_2 = 100% (P_AO_2 = 673 mm Hg).
Calculate the end-capillary oxygen content (C_cO_2).

(A) 20.1 vol%
(B) 21.4 vol%
(C) 22.1 vol%
(D) 23.2 vol%

Handwritten: $15 \times 1.34 \times 100$
20.1 + 2.03 = 22.119%
2.019

57d. Which of the following measurements has the highest calculated end-capillary oxygen content (C_cO_2)?

	Hb (g%)	F_IO_2 (%)	P_AO_2 (mm Hg)
(A)	15	21	100
(B)	12	80	530
(C)	11	100	673
(D)	14	40	235

57e. A polycythemic patient who is recovering from coronary artery bypass surgery has the following measurements: Hb = 17 g%, F_IO_2 = 30% (P_AO_2 = 164 mm Hg). What is the calculated C_cO_2 for this patient?

(A) 20.1 vol%
(B) 21.9 vol%
(C) 22.8 vol%
(D) 23.3 vol%

Handwritten: $17 \times 1.34 =$ $164 \times 0.003 = 0.492$
22.78

= 23.272

Chapter

58

Oxygen Content: Mixed Venous ($C_{\bar{v}}O_2$)

NOTE

Mixed venous oxygen content ($C_{\bar{v}}O_2$) reflects the overall oxygen level of the blood returning to the right heart. $C_{\bar{v}}O_2$ is affected by a number of factors. Low Hb level (e.g., anemia), low O_2 saturation (e.g., hypoxemia), decrease in cardiac output (e.g., congestive heart failure), or increase in metabolic rate (e.g., exercise) significantly lower the $C_{\bar{v}}O_2$. Refer to Table 2-7 for factors that decrease the mixed venous oxygen content.

EQUATION

$$C_{\bar{v}}O_2 = (Hb \times 1.34 \times S_{\bar{v}}O_2) + (P_{\bar{v}}O_2 \times 0.003)$$

$C_{\bar{v}}O_2$: Mixed venous oxygen content in vol%
Hb : Hemoglobin content in g%
1.34 : Amount of oxygen that 1 g of fully saturated hemoglobin can hold
$S_{\bar{v}}O_2$: Mixed venous oxygen saturation in vol%
$P_{\bar{v}}O_2$: Mixed venous oxygen tension mm Hg

0.003 : Amount of dissolved oxygen for 1 mm HG of P_aO_2

NORMAL VALUE

12 to 15 vol%

EXAMPLE

Given: Hb = 15 g%
$S_{\bar{v}}O_2$ = 70%
$P_{\bar{v}}O_2$ = 35 mm Hg
Calculate the mixed venous oxygen content ($C_{\bar{v}}O_2$).
$$\begin{aligned} C_{\bar{v}}O_2 &= (Hb \times 1.34 \times S_{\bar{v}}O_2) + (P_{\bar{v}}O_2 \times 0.003) \\ &= (15 \times 1.34 \times 70\%) + (35 \times 0.003) \\ &= 14.07 + 0.11 \\ &= 14.18 \text{ vol}\% \end{aligned}$$

EXERCISE

Given: Hb = 12 g%
$S_{\bar{v}}O_2$ = 75%
$P_{\bar{v}}O_2$ = 40 mm Hg
Calculate the $C_{\bar{v}}O_2$.

[Answer: $C_{\bar{v}}O_2$ = 12.18 vol%]

REFERENCES

Burton; Shapiro

TABLE 2-7. Factors That Decrease $C_{\bar{v}}O_2$

Low hemoglobin

Low O_2 saturation

Decreased cardiac output

Increased metabolic rate

SEE *Oxygen Content: Arterial (C_aO_2); Oxygen Content: End-Capillary (C_cO_2).*

SELF-ASSESSMENT QUESTIONS

58a. Given: Hb = 13 g%, $S_{\bar{v}}O_2$ = 70%, $P_{\bar{v}}O_2$ = 40 mm Hg. Calculate the mixed venous oxygen content ($C_{\bar{v}}O_2$).

(A) 12.3 vol%

(B) 12.9 vol%

(C) 13.6 vol%

(D) 14.2 vol%

58b. A sample obtained from the pulmonary artery has the following results: Hb = 14 g%, $S_{\bar{v}}O_2$ = 75%, $P_{\bar{v}}O_2$ = 40 mm Hg. Calculate the $C_{\bar{v}}O_2$. Is it normal?

(A) 12.3 vol%; abnormal

(B) 13.6 vol%; normal

(C) 13.6 vol%; abnormal

(D) 14.2 vol%; normal

58c. Which of the following blood gas measurements has the lowest mixed venous oxygen content ($C_{\bar{v}}O_2$)?

	Hb (g%)	$S_{\bar{v}}O_2$ (%)	$P_{\bar{v}}O_2$ (mm Hg)
(A)	13	74	30
(B)	15	66	34
(C)	14	75	38
(D)	14	72	36

58d. An anemic patient who is admitted for shortness of breath has the following measurements: Hb = 9 g%, $S_{\bar{v}}O_2$ = 73%; $P_{\bar{v}}O_2$ = 38 mm Hg. What is the calculated $C_{\bar{v}}O_2$ for this patient? Is it normal?

(A) 8.9 vol%; abnormal

(B) 8.9 vol%; normal

(C) 12.1 vol%; abnormal

(D) 12.1 vol%; normal

Chapter

59

Oxygen Duration of E Cylinder

NOTES

In this type of oxygen duration calculation, it is essential to remember the conversion factor (0.28) for the E oxygen cylinder (Appendix E). This conversion factor (0.28 L/psig) is derived by dividing the volume of oxygen (622 L) by the gauge pressure (2,200 psig) of a full E cylinder (622 L/2,200 psig = 0.283 L/psig).

The 622 L comes from 22 ft^3 × 28.3 L/ft^3 as an E cylinder holds about 22 ft^3 of compressed oxygen and each ft^3 of compressed oxygen gives 28.3 L of gaseous oxygen.

To change minutes to hours and minutes, simply divide the minutes by 60. The whole number represents the hours, and the remainder is the minutes.

When a calculator is used, the number in front of the decimal is the hours. The number after the decimal, including the decimal point, should be multiplied by 60 to obtain minutes.

EQUATION

$$\text{Duration of E} = \frac{0.28 \times \text{psig}}{\text{Liter flow}}$$

Duration of E : Duration of oxygen remaining in an E cylinder in minutes

psig : Gauge pressure, in pounds per square inch (psi)

Liter flow : Oxygen flow rate in L/min

EXAMPLE

Given: E oxygen cylinder with 2,000 psig
Oxygen flow = 5 L/min

A. Calculate how long the cylinder will last until 0 psig.

$$\begin{aligned}
\text{Duration} &= \frac{0.28 \times \text{psig}}{\text{Liter flow}} \\
&= \frac{0.28 \times 2,000}{5} \\
&= \frac{560}{5} \\
&= 112 \text{ min or 1 hr 52 min}
\end{aligned}$$

B. Calculate how long the cylinder will last until the pressure reaches 500 psig.

$$\begin{aligned}
\text{Duration to 500 psig} &= \frac{0.28 \times (\text{psig} - 500)}{\text{Liter flow}} \\
&= \frac{0.28 \times (2,000 - 500)}{5} \\
&= \frac{0.28 \times 1,500}{5} \\
&= \frac{420}{5} \\
&= 84 \text{ min or 1 hr 24 min}
\end{aligned}$$

EXERCISE 1

Given: E oxygen cylinder with 2,200 psig
Oxygen flow rate = 5 L/min

How long will the oxygen remain in this cylinder at this flow rate until the cylinder reaches 0 psig?

[Answer: Duration = 123 min or 2 hr 3 min]

EXERCISE 2

Given: E oxygen cylinder with 1,600 psig
Oxygen flow rate = 2 L/min
Calculate the duration of oxygen remaining in this cylinder (to 0 psig). How long will it last until 500 psig?

[Answer: Duration = 224 min or 3 hr 44 min

Duration to 500 psig = 154 min or 2 hr 34 min]

REFERENCES

White; Wilkins (2)

SELF-ASSESSMENT QUESTIONS

59a. Given: E oxygen cylinder with 2,000 psig, oxygen flow = 2 L/min. Calculate the duration until the pressure reaches 0 psig at this flow rate.

(A) 3 hr 55 min
(B) 4 hr 15 min
(C) 4 hr 30 min
(D) 4 hr 40 min

59b. An E oxygen cylinder is full at 2,200 psig. If a flow rate is set at 2 L/min, how long will this cylinder last until it reaches a gauge pressure of 200 psig?

(A) 1 hr 20 min
(B) 3 hr 30 min
(C) 4 hr 40 min
(D) 5 hr 10 min

59c. An E oxygen cylinder with 1,400 psig is available for patient transport. At an oxygen flow rate of 2 L/min, what is the maximum travel time the patient can rely on until this cylinder reaches 500 psig?

(A) 1 hr
(B) 1 hr 10 min
(C) 2 hr 6 min
(D) 3 hr 16 min

59d. An E oxygen cylinder with 1,800 psig is being used at a flow rate of 3 L/min. How long will the cylinder last until the pressure reaches 0 psig? Until the pressure reaches 200 psig?

(A) 2 hr 48 min; 2 hr 29 min
(B) 2 hr 48 min; 2 hr 10 min
(C) 3 hr 20 min; 3 hr 1 min
(D) 3 hr 20 min; 2 hr 42 min

59e. At its respective flow rate, which of the following E cylinders would provide the longest duration of oxygen?

	psig	Flow (L/min)
(A)	500	1
(B)	700	1.5
(C)	800	2
(D)	900	2.5

60

Oxygen Duration
of H or K Cylinder

NOTES

In this type of oxygen duration calculation, it is essential to remember the conversion factor (3.14) for the H or K oxygen cylinder (Appendix E). This conversion factor (3.14 L/psig) is derived by dividing the volume of oxygen (6,900 L) by the gauge pressure (2,200 psig) of a full H or K cylinder:

$$\frac{6900 \text{ L}}{2200 \text{ psig}} = 3.136 \text{ L/psig}$$

The 6900 L comes from 224 ft^3 × 28.3 L/ft^3 because H and K cylinders hold about 244 ft^3 of compressed oxygen, and each ft^3 of compressed oxygen gives 28.3 L of gaseous oxygen.

To change minutes to hours and minutes, simply divide the minutes by 60. The whole number represents the hours, and the remainder is the minutes.

When a calculator is used to divide, the number in front of the decimal is the hours. The number after the decimal, including the decimal point, should be multiplied by 60 to obtain minutes.

EQUATION

$$\text{Duration of H or K} = \frac{3.14 \times \text{psig}}{\text{Liter flow}}$$

Duration of H or K : Duration of oxygen remaining in an H or K cylinder in minutes

psig : Gauge pressure, pounds per square inch (psi)

Liter flow : Oxygen flow rate in L/min

EXAMPLE

Given: Size H oxygen cylinder with 1,000 psig
     Oxygen flow = 5 L/min

A. Calculate how long the cylinder will last until 0 psig.

$$
\begin{aligned}
\text{Duration} &= \frac{3.14 \times \text{psig}}{\text{Liter flow}} \\
&= \frac{3.14 \times 1,000}{5} \\
&= \frac{3,140}{5} \\
&= 628 \text{ min or } 10 \text{ hr } 28 \text{ min}
\end{aligned}
$$

B. Calculate how long the cylinder will last until the pressure reaches 200 psig.

$$
\begin{aligned}
\text{Duration to 200 psig} &= \frac{3.14 \times (\text{psig} - 200)}{\text{Liter flow}} \\
&= \frac{3.14 \times (1,000 - 200)}{5} \\
&= \frac{3.14 \times 800}{5} \\
&= \frac{2,512}{5} \\
&= 502 \text{ min or } 8 \text{ hr } 22 \text{ min}
\end{aligned}
$$

EXERCISE

Given: Size K oxygen cylinder with 2,200 psig
         Oxygen flow rate = 2 L/min
Calculate the duration of oxygen remaining in this cylinder.
How long will the cylinder last until it reaches 200 psig?

[Answer: Duration = 3,454 min or 57 hr 34 min;

Duration to 200 psig = 3,140 min or 52 hr 20 min]

REFERENCES

White; Wilkins (2)

SELF-ASSESSMENT QUESTIONS

60a. An H oxygen cylinder has a gauge pressure of 1,600 psig and is running at a flow rate of 5 L/min. How long will it take the pressure to reach 0 psig at this flow rate?

(A) 12 hr 10 min
(B) 14 hr 20 min
(C) 16 hr 45 min
(D) 18 hr 55 min

60b. Given: K oxygen cylinder with 2,200 psig, oxygen flow = 5 L/min. Calculate the duration until the pressure reaches 0 psig at this flow rate.

(A) 2 hr
(B) 22 hr
(C) 23 hr
(D) 24 hr

60c. Given: H oxygen cylinder with 1,200 psig, oxygen flow rate = 2 L/min. Calculate the duration of oxygen remaining in this cylinder until it reaches 200 psig.

(A) 16 hr 15 min
(B) 18 hr
(C) 20 hr 30 min
(D) 26 hr 10 min

60d. A K oxygen cylinder has a gauge reading of 1,700 psig. How long will this cylinder last until it reaches 500 psig at an oxygen flow rate of 2 L/min?

(A) 30 hr 16 min
(B) 31 hr 24 min
(C) 32 hr 10 min
(D) 33 hr 42 min

60e. An H oxygen cylinder with 2,000 psig is being used at a flow rate of 3 L/min. How long will the cylinder last until the pressure reaches 0 psig? Until the pressure reaches 500 psig?

(A) 29 hr 35 min; 18 hr 8 min
(B) 29 hr 35 min; 21 hr 12 min
(C) 34 hr 53 min; 24 hr 26 min
(D) 34 hr 53 min; 26 hr 10 min

60f. During the last oxygen rounds at 10 P.M., an H oxygen cylinder has a gauge reading of 800 psig and the oxygen flow was set at 5 L/min. At this oxygen flow rate, about what time the next morning will the gauge reading reach 500 psig?

(A) 1 A.M.

(B) 2 A.M.

(C) 3 A.M.

(D) 6 A.M.

60g. Which of the following H cylinders would provide the longest duration of oxygen at its respective oxygen flow rate?

	psig	Flow (L/min)
(A)	600	2
(B)	700	2.5
(C)	800	3
(D)	900	3.5

Chapter

61

Oxygen Duration of Liquid System

In this type of oxygen duration calculation, it is essential to remember the conversion factor (344 L/lb) for the liquid oxygen cylinders. This conversion factor comes from 860/2.5 = 344 (Figure 2-38). Liquid oxygen expands about 860 times to become gaseous oxygen, and it weighs 2.5 lb/L.

If the net weight of liquid oxygen is not shown, one can compute it by weighing the cylinder and liquid oxygen and subtracting the weight of the empty cylinder.

To change minutes to hours and minutes, simply divide minutes by 60. The whole number represents the hours, and the remainder is the minutes.

When a calculator is used to divide, the number in front of the decimal is the hours. The number after the decimal, including the decimal point, should be multiplied by 60 to get minutes.

The calculated duration does not account for the amount of liquid oxygen lost by normal evaporation. The evaporative rate of liquid oxygen ranges from 1 to 1.8 lb (0.4 to 0.72 liquid liters or 344 to 619 gaseous liters) per day.

EQUATION 1

> When the liquid weight is known:

$$\text{Duration} = \frac{344 \times \text{Liquid weight}}{\text{Flow}}$$

Duration : Duration of oxygen remaining in a *liquid* O_2 cylinder, in min

344 : A conversion factor, in L/lb

Liquid weight : The *net weight* of liquid oxygen in lb

Flow : Oxygen flow rate in L/min

EXAMPLE 1

If the net weight of liquid oxygen in a cylinder is 2 lb and the patient is using the contents at 1 L/min, how long will the liquid oxygen last?

$$\text{Duration} = \frac{344 \times \text{Liquid weight}}{\text{Flow}}$$

$$= \frac{344 \times 2}{1}$$

$$= \frac{688}{1}$$

$$= 688 \text{ min or } 11 \text{ hr } 28 \text{ min}$$

EXERCISE

If the net weight of liquid oxygen in a cylinder is 2.5 lb, how long will the liquid oxygen last if the oxygen flow is running at 2 L/min?

[Answer: Duration = 430 min or 7 hr 10 min]

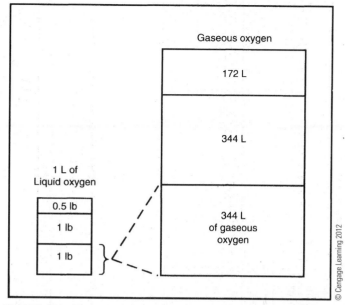

Figure 2-37 Volume relationship of liquid and gaseous oxygen. One liter of liquid oxygen weighs about 2.5 lbs. One pound of liquid oxygen equals 344 L of gaseous oxygen.

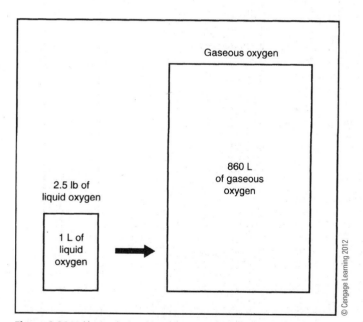

Figure 2-38 Volume relationship of liquid and gaseous oxygen. One liter of liquid oxygen weighs about 2.5 lbs and is equal to 860 L of gaseous oxygen.

NOTES

One liter of liquid oxygen expands to about 860 L of gaseous oxygen (Figure 2-38). Therefore, the liquid capacity is converted to gaseous capacity by multiplying the liquid capacity by 860.

To change minutes to hours and minutes, simply divide minutes by 60. The whole number represents the hours, and the remainder is the minutes.

When a calculator is used to divide, the number in front of the decimal is the hours. The number after the decimal, including the decimal point, should be multiplied by 60 to get minutes.

The calculated duration does not account for the amount of liquid oxygen lost by normal evaporation. The evaporative rate of liquid oxygen ranges from 1 to 1.8 lb (0.4 to 0.72 liquid liters of 344 to 619 gaseous liters) per day.

EQUATION 2

> When the gauge fraction is known:

$$\text{Duration} = \frac{\text{Capacity} \times 860 \times \text{Gauge fraction}}{\text{Flow}}$$

Duration	:	Duration of oxygen remaining in a *liquid* O_2 cylinder, in min
Capacity	:	Capacity of liquid oxygen in cylinder, in L
860	:	Factor to convert liquid to gaseous oxygen, in L
Gauge fraction	:	Fractional reading of cylinder content
Flow	:	Oxygen flow rate in L/min

EXAMPLE 2

A portable liquid oxygen cylinder has a liquid capacity of 0.60 L. What is the gaseous capacity?

$$\begin{aligned}
\text{Gaseous capacity} &= \text{Liquid capacity} \times 860 \\
&= 0.60 \times 860 \\
&= 516 \text{ L}
\end{aligned}$$

EXAMPLE 3

If the capacity of a liquid oxygen cylinder is 2.0 L and the gauge reading of the cylinder indicates it is $\frac{1}{3}$ full, how long will the liquid oxygen last if the flow is at 2 L/min?

$$\begin{aligned}
\text{Duration} &= \frac{\text{Capacity} \times 860 \times \text{Gauge fraction}}{\text{Flow}} \\
&= \frac{2 \times 860 \times \frac{1}{3}}{2} \\
&= \frac{1,720 \times \frac{1}{3}}{2} \\
&= \frac{573}{2} \\
&= 287 \text{ min or 4 hr 47 min}
\end{aligned}$$

EXERCISE

If the capacity of a liquid oxygen cylinder is 1.8 L and the gauge reading indicates it is $\frac{1}{2}$ full, how long will the liquid oxygen last if the oxygen flow is at 1 L/min?

[Answer: Duration = 774 min or 12 hr 54 min]

REFERENCE

Wilkins (2)

SELF-ASSESSMENT QUESTIONS

61a. One pound of liquid oxygen can be expanded to become how many liters of gaseous oxygen?

(A) 2.5 L
(B) 344 L
(C) 500 L
(D) 860 L

61b. One liter of liquid oxygen weighs _____ pounds, and each liter can be expanded to become _____ liters of gaseous oxygen.

    (A) 2 lb; 100 L

    (B) 2 lb; 344 L

    (C) 2.5 lb; 500 L

    (D) 2.5 lb; 860 L

61c. Given: net weight of liquid oxygen in a cylinder = 4 lb. How long will the liquid oxygen last if the oxygen flow rate is 2 L/min?

    (A) 6 hr 33 min

    (B) 8 hr

    (C) 10 hr

    (D) 11 hr 28 min

61d. The net weight of liquid oxygen in a cylinder is 3 lb. If a patient is using 2 L/min of oxygen on a continuous basis, how long will the liquid oxygen last?

    (A) 7 hr 43 min

    (B) 7 hr 50 min

    (C) 8 hr 6 min

    (D) 8 hr 36 min

61e. A portable liquid oxygen cylinder has a net weight of 1.5 lb. At a flow rate of 1.5 L/min of oxygen, how long will it last until the portable system needs refilling?

    (A) 4 hr 23 min

    (B) 4 hr 45 min

    (C) 5 hr 44 min

    (D) 6 hr 30 min

61f. The net weight remaining in a stationary liquid oxygen system is 10 lb, and the home care patient is using it 8 hr per day during sleep at a flow rate of 1 L/min. Based on this usage, about how many days will this liquid oxygen system last?

    (A) 6 days

    (B) 7 days

    (C) 8 days

    (D) 9 days

61g. If the capacity of a full liquid oxygen cylinder is 0.42 L, how long will the liquid oxygen last at a flow rate of 1 L/min?

    (A) 6 hr 1 min

    (B) 7 hr 16 min

    (C) 8 hr

    (D) 9 hr 25 min

61h. A portable liquid oxygen cylinder has a liquid capacity of 0.49 L. What is the gaseous capacity?

(A) 387 L

(B) 403 L

(C) 421 L

(D) 452 L

61i. The capacity of a portable liquid oxygen cylinder is 2 L, and the gauge reading indicates it is $\frac{1}{2}$ full. If a patient is using 2 L/min of oxygen on a continuous basis, how long will the liquid oxygen last?

(A) 7 hr 10 min

(B) 7 hr 45 min

(C) 8 hr 36 min

(D) 9 hr 24 min

61j. The capacity of a stationary home liquid oxygen system is 25.5 L, and it is $\frac{1}{4}$ full. If a patient is using 1.5 L/min of oxygen on a continuous basis, about how many hours will his liquid system last?

(A) 40 hr

(B) 50 hr

(C) 60 hr

(D) 70 hr

61k. The liquid capacity of a full stationary liquid oxygen system is 37 L, and the home care patient is using it 8 hr per day during sleep at a flow rate of 2 L/min. Based on this usage, about how many days will this liquid oxygen system last?

(A) 11 days

(B) 22 days

(C) 33 days

(D) 44 days

Chapter

62

Oxygen Extraction Ratio (O$_2$ER)

NOTES

Oxygen extraction ratio (O$_2$ER) is also known as the oxygen utilization ratio or oxygen coefficient ratio. In the O$_2$ER equation, C_aO_2 represents the total amount of oxygen available for peripheral tissue utilization, and $C_aO_2 - C_{\bar{v}}O_2$ reflects the amount of oxygen extracted or consumed by the peripheral tissues.

The O$_2$ER provides a useful indication of a patient's oxygen transport status. Factors that cause a low C_aO_2 or a high $C(a-\bar{v})O_2$ lead to a high O$_2$ER value. On the other hand, factors that contribute to a high C_aO_2 or a low $C(a-\bar{v})O_2$ result in a low O$_2$ER value. Tables 2-8 and 2-9 summarize the major factors that affect the oxygen extraction ratio.

EQUATION

$$O_2ER = \frac{C_aO_2 - C_{\bar{v}}O_2}{C_aO_2}$$

O$_2$ER : Oxygen extraction ratio in %
C_aO_2 : Arterial oxygen content in vol%
$C_{\bar{v}}O_2$: Mixed venous oxygen content in vol%

NORMAL VALUE

20 to 28%

EXAMPLE

Given: C_aO_2 = 20 vol%
$\quad\quad\quad C_{\bar{v}}O_2$ = 16 vol%
What is the calculated oxygen extraction ratio (O$_2$ER)?

$$O_2ER = \frac{C_aO_2 - C_{\bar{v}}O_2}{C_aO_2}$$

$$= \frac{20 - 16}{20}$$

$$= \frac{4}{20}$$

$$= 0.2 \text{ or } 20\%$$

TABLE 2-8. Factors That Increase the O$_2$ER

Decreased cardiac output

Periods of increased oxygen consumption

  Exercise

  Seizures

  Shivering in postoperative patient

  Hyperthermia

Anemia

Decreased arterial oxygenation

TABLE 2-9. Factors That Decrease the O_2ER

Increased cardiac output

Peripheral shunting (e.g., sepsis, trauma)

Certain poisons (e.g., cyanide prevents cellular metabolism)

Hypothermia (slows cellular metabolism)

Increased hemoglobin concentration

Increased arterial oxygenation

EXERCISE

What is the calculated oxygen extraction ratio (O_2ER) for a patient with the following oxygen contents:

$C_aO_2 = 19$ vol%
$C_{\bar{v}}O_2 = 16$ vol%

[Answer: O_2ER = 15.8%]

REFERENCE

Des Jardins

SEE

Appendix V: Oxygen Transport Normal Ranges.

SELF-ASSESSMENT QUESTIONS

62a. Given: $C_aO_2 = 21$ vol%, $C_{\bar{v}}O_2 = 16.5$ vol%. Calculate the oxygen extraction ratio (O_2ER).

(A) 4.5%
(B) 16.5%
(C) 21%
(D) 79%

62b. For a patient with these oxygen contents: $C_aO_2 = 20.4$ vol%, $C_{\bar{v}}O_2 = 15.6$ vol%, what is the calculated oxygen extraction ratio (O_2ER)?

(A) 4.8%
(B) 15.6%
(C) 20.4%
(D) 23.5%

62c. Which of the following pairs of oxygen content measurements has the highest oxygen extraction ratio?

	C_aO_2 (vol%)	$C_{\bar{v}}O_2$ (vol%)
(A)	21	16
(B)	21	17
(C)	20	16
(D)	20	17

62d. Which of the following pairs of oxygen content measurements
has the lowest oxygen extraction ratio?

	C_aO_2 (vol%)	$C_{\bar{v}}O_2$ (vol%)
(A)	18.5	13.8
(B)	18.5	14.2
(C)	19.3	14.2
(D)	19.3	15.5

Chapter

63

Partial Pressure of a Dry Gas

NOTES

Dalton's law states that the partial pressures of all gases in a gas mixture equal the total pressure exerted by the gas mixture. Therefore, the partial pressure of a gas can be determined by multiplying the barometric pressure (P_B) by the percentage of the gas in the mixture ($\%_g$).

At high altitude, the P_B decreases, and consequently the partial pressures of all gases also decrease. For example, at an altitude of 26,000 ft above sea level (P_B = 270 mm Hg), PO_2 = 270 mm Hg × 0.21 = 56.7 mm Hg. On the other hand, hyperbaric conditions (e.g., below sea level, hyperbaric chambers) increase the barometric pressure and partial pressures of all gases. At a depth of 66 ft below sea level (P_B = 2,280 mm Hg), PO_2 = 2,280 mm Hg × 0.21 = 478.8 mm Hg.

Under normal clinical conditions, the barometric pressure varies very little. By increasing the percentage of a gas (oxygen concentration), a higher partial pressure of that gas may be achieved. This is the basis of oxygen therapy.

EQUATION

$P_g = P_B \times \%_g$
P_g : Partial pressure of a dry gas
P_B : Barometric pressure in mm Hg
$\%_g$: Percent of gas in the mixture

EXAMPLE

What is the partial pressure of (a) nitrogen and (b) oxygen in an air sample at a barometric pressure of 720 mm Hg?
As nitrogen comprises 78% of air:
A. $PN_2 = P_B \times \%N_2$
   $= 720 \times 78\%$
   $= 561.6$ mm Hg
As oxygen comprises 21% of air:
B. $PO_2 = P_B \times \%0_2$
   $= 720 \times 21\%$
   $= 151.2$ mm Hg

EXERCISE

Calculate the partial pressure of oxygen in a dry air sample at 40,000 ft above sea level (P_B = 141 mm Hg). (F_IO_2 at 40,000 ft above sea level = 21%.)

[Answer: PO_2 = 29.6 mm Hg]

REFERENCE

Wilkins (2)

SEE

Alveolar Oxygen Tension (P_AO_2); Dalton's Law of Partial Pressure; Appendix C: Barometric Pressures at Selected Altitudes.

SELF-ASSESSMENT QUESTIONS

63a. At sea level (P_B = 760 mm Hg), what is the partial pressure of oxygen in a dry, ambient air sample?

   (A) 100 mm Hg
   (B) 115 mm Hg
   (C) 126 mm Hg
   (D) 159 mm Hg

63b. At 33 ft below sea level (P_B = 1,520 mm Hg), what is the partial
pressure of oxygen of a diver's inspired air?

(A) 286 mm Hg
(B) 319 mm Hg
(C) 371 mm Hg
(D) 425 mm Hg

$1,520 \times 0.21 = 0.3192$

63c. Calculate the partial pressure of oxygen in a dry air sample at
10,000 ft above sea level (P_B = 523 mm Hg).

(A) 80 mm Hg
(B) 94 mm Hg
(C) 110 mm Hg
(D) 122 mm Hg

$523 \times 0.21 = 109.83$

63d. Carbon dioxide makes up 0.03% of ambient air. Calculate its
partial pressure in a dry air sample at sea level (P_B = 760 mm Hg).

(A) 0.23 mm Hg
(B) 2.28 mm Hg
(C) 22.8 mm Hg
(D) 228 mm Hg

$760 \times 0.03\% = 22.8$

Chapter

64

PCO_2 to H_2CO_3

NOTES

In the Henderson-Hasselbalch equation, the carbonic acid (H_2CO_3) concentration is represented by the solubility coefficient (0.03) times the partial pressure of arterial carbon dioxide (P_aCO_2).

H_2CO_3 is an important factor in acid-base balance because of its role in determining the blood pH. As the denominator of the Henderson-Hasselbalch equation, H_2CO_3 (P_aCO_2) is inversely related to the pH. In other words, a high H_2CO_3 (P_aCO_2) level with normal HCO_3^- results in a low pH (acidosis). A low H_2CO_3 (P_aCO_2) level with normal HCO_3^- results in a high pH (alkalosis).

Note also that the conversion factor used for P_aCO_2 to H_2CO_3 is 0.03 and the conversion factor for PO_2 to oxygen content is 0.003. These two factors look similar and must be used with care.

EQUATION

$H_2CO_3 = P_aCO_2 \times 0.03$
H_2CO_3 : Carbonate acid in mEq/L
P_aCO_2 : Arterial carbon dioxide tension in mm Hg

NORMAL VALUE

1.05 to 1.35 mEq/L

EXAMPLE

Given: $P_aCO_2 = 40$ mm Hg
What is the calculated carbonic acid level?
$H_2CO_3 = P_aCO_2 \times 0.03$
$\quad\quad\quad = 40 \times 0.03$
$\quad\quad\quad = 1.2$ mEq/L

EXERCISE

Given: $P_aCO_2 = 50$ mm Hg
Calculate the H_2CO_3 level.

[Answer: $H_2CO_3 = 1.5$ mEq/L]

REFERENCE

Shapiro

SEE

pH (Henderson-Hasselbalch).

SELF-ASSESSMENT QUESTIONS

64a. The amount of carbonic acid can be determined by using the equation:

(A) $0.003 \times P_aCO_2$.

(B) $0.03 \times P_aCO_2$.

(C) $0.3 \times P_aCO_2$.

(D) $pK + \log \dfrac{HCO_3^-}{H_2CO_3}$.

64b. Based on the pH equation, a P_aCO$_2$ of 50 mm Hg equals _____ mEq/L of carbonic acid.

(A) 1.5

(B) 1.2

(C) 1.0

(D) 0.5

64c. A blood gas measurement shows that the P_aCO$_2$ is 30 mm Hg. What is the calculated carbonic acid level?

(A) 0.15 mEq/L

(B) 1.5 mEq/L

(C) 15 mEq/L

(D) 0.9 mEq/L

64d. Which of the following P_aCO$_2$ values corresponds with a carbonic acid level of 1.2 mEq/L?

(A) 20 mm Hg

(B) 30 mm Hg

(C) 40 mm Hg

(D) 50 mm Hg

Chapter

65

pH (Henderson-Hasselbalch)

NOTES

The pH value is directly related to the bicarbonate (HCO_3^-) level, and it is inversely related to the carbonic acid (H_2CO_3) or the carbon dioxide tension (PCO_2) level.

Unless there is compensation, the pH will be greater than 7.40 with an increase of HCO_3^- (metabolic alkalosis) or a decrease of PCO_2 (respiratory alkalosis). In other words, if the HCO_3^- : H_2CO_3 ratio is *greater than 20:1*, the pH will be *higher than 7.40*.

On the other hand, the pH will be less than 7.40 with a decrease of HCO_3^- (metabolic acidosis) or an increase of PCO_2 (respiratory acidosis). In other words, if the HCO_3^- : H_2CO_3 ratio is *less than 20:1*, the pH will be *lower than 7.40*.

It is essential to note that the pH will be 7.40 as long as the HCO_3^-:H_2CO_3 ratio is 20:1. The Example and Exercise 1 illustrate this compensatory effect even though the HCO_3^- and PCO_2 values are quite different in these two cases.

EQUATION 1

$$pH = 6.1 + \log\left[\frac{HCO_3^-}{H_2CO_3}\right]$$

EQUATION 2

$$pH = 6.1 + \log\left[\frac{HCO_3^-}{PCO_2 \times 0.03}\right]$$

pH   : Puissance hydrogen, negative logarithm of H^+ ion concentration

HCO_3^- : Serum bicarbonate concentration in mEq/L
H_2CO_3 : Carbonate acid in mEq/L
PCO_2 : Carbon dioxide tension in mm Hg

NORMAL VALUE

Arterial pH   = 7.40 (7.35 to 7.45)
Mixed venous pH = 7.36

EXAMPLE

Given: $H_2CO_3^-$: 24 mEq/L
          PCO_2 : 40 mm Hg
Calculate the pH.

$$pH = 6.1 + \log\left[\frac{HCO_3^-}{PCO_2 \times 0.03}\right]$$

$$= 6.1 + \log\left[\frac{24}{40 \times 0.03}\right]$$

$$= 6.1 + \log\left[\frac{24}{1.2}\right]$$

$$= 6.1 + \log 20$$

(From the common logarithms of numbers in Appendix S, log 20 = 1.301.)
pH = 6.1 + 1.301
    = 7.401 or 7.40

EXERCISE 1

Given: HCO_3^- = 30 mEq/L
         PCO_2 = 50 mm Hg
         log 20 = 1.301
Calculate the pH.

[Answer: pH = 7.401 or 7.40]

EXERCISE 2   Given: $HCO_3^- = 16$ mEq/L
$PCO_2 = 32$ mm Hg
Use the Henderson-Hasselbalch equation and common logarithms of numbers in Appendix S to calculate the pH.

[Answer: pH = 7.32 as log 16.67 = 1.222]

REFERENCES   Shapiro; Wojciechowski

SEE   *Appendix S: Logarithm Table.*

SELF-ASSESSMENT QUESTIONS

65a. When the ratio of bicarbonate to carbonic acid in blood is 20:1, the pH is:

(A) 6.80.
(B) 7.20.
(C) 7.40.
(D) 7.60.

65b. The pH is normal (7.40) when the bicarbonate to carbonic acid ratio is:

(A) 20 : 1.
(B) 24 : 1.
(C) 1 : 20.
(D) 1 : 24.

65c. Given: $HCO_3^- = 30$ mEq/L, $PCO_2 = 50$ mm Hg. The calculated pH is about:

(A) 7.20.
(B) 7.25.
(C) 7.35.
(D) 7.40.

65d. At a pH of 7.50, the ratio of bicarbonate to carbonic acid in blood is about:

(A) 10 : 1.
(B) 20 : 1.
(C) 26 : 1.
(D) 35 : 1.

65e. From the logarithm table in Appendix S, find the value of log 20.

(A) 0.30
(B) 3.00
(C) 30.0
(D) 1.30

65f. From the logarithm table in Appendix S, find the value of log 16.

(A) 0.3

(B) 1.2

(C) 2.04

(D) 3

65g. Given: $HCO_3^- = 34$ mEq/L, $PCO_2 = 65$ mm Hg. Which of the following is used to calculate the pH? What is the calculated pH?

(A) $6.1 + \log 17.4$; 7.34

(B) $6.1 + \log 19.1$; 7.38

(C) $6.1 + \log 20.1$; 7.40

(D) $\log 19.1$; 7.38

65h. Use the logarithm table in Appendix S to calculate the pH if the HCO_3^- level is 16 mEq/L and $PCO_2 = 60$ mm Hg. Is the pH normal or abnormal?

(A) 7.05; normal

(B) 7.05; abnormal

(C) 7.11; normal

(D) 7.11; abnormal

65i. Which of the following is *incorrect* with regard to the pH (Henderson-Hasselbalch) equation?

(A) The pH is directly related to the HCO_3^- level.

(B) The pH is inversely related to the PCO_2 level.

(C) The pH will be 7.40 if the HCO_3^- to H_2CO_3 ratio is 20:1.

(D) The pH will be greater than 7.40 if the HCO_3^- to PCO_2 ratio is less than 20:1.

Chapter

66

Poiseuille Equation

The Poiseuille equation describes the characteristic of flow (turbulent or laminar) in the airway. It is influenced by the driving pressure difference, gas viscosity, and radius and length of the airway.

The abbreviated equation shows the inverse relationship between the work of breathing (ΔP) and radius of airway (r).

EQUATION

$$\dot{V} = \frac{\Delta P r^4 \pi}{\mu l 8}$$

$\dot{V}$: Flow
ΔP : Driving pressure
r : Radius of airway
$\dfrac{\pi}{8}$: Constant for equation
μ : Viscosity of gas
l : Length of airway

Under clinical conditions where viscosity of gas (μ), length of airway (l), and $\pi/8$ remain stable and unchanged, they may be deleted in order to look at the relationship among the remaining variables of the equation. The abbreviated form of the Poiseuille equation is as follows:

$$\Delta P = \frac{\dot{V}}{r^4}$$

This equation shows that when the radius of the airway (r) decreases by half, the driving pressure (ΔP) must increase 16 times to maintain the same flow. In other words, bronchoconstriction (decrease in r) can cause a tremendously large increase in the work of breathing (increase in ΔP). If the work of breathing cannot keep up with the bronchoconstriction, air flow ($\dot{V}$) will be decreased. In pulmonary function testing, reduction in flow rate measurements is generally indicative of bronchoconstriction.

REFERENCE

White

SELF-ASSESSMENT QUESTIONS

66a. Which of the following is the simplified form of the Poiseuille equation describing the relationship between work of breathing and radius of airway?

(A) $\Delta P = \dot{V} \times r^2$

(B) $\Delta P = \dfrac{\dot{V}}{r^2}$

(C) $\Delta P = \dot{V} \times r^4$

(D) $\Delta P = \dfrac{\dot{V}}{r^4}$

66b. _____ shows that the size of the airway is directly related to the gas flow and inversely related to the work of breathing.

(A) Henry's law
(B) Law of LaPlace
(C) Poiseuille equation
(D) Law of Continuity

66c. The Poiseuille equation shows that when the radius of the airway (r) decreases by half, the driving pressure (ΔP) must increase _____ times to maintain the same flow rate.

(A) 4
(B) 8
(C) 16
(D) 32

66d. Bronchoconstriction can cause a very large increase in the work of breathing because of the changes in the _____ of the airway.

(A) cilia
(B) mucosa
(C) radius
(D) length

Chapter

67

Predicted P_aO_2 Based on Age

NOTES

This equation is used to estimate the P_aO_2 value of a healthy person breathing room air. The predicted P_aO_2 decreases with age.

In Sorbini et al., the predicted P_aO_2 in healthy subjects declines by 0.43 mm Hg per year of age.

If the patient is in a semi-Fowler position, use the P_aO_2 (seated) equation.

EQUATION 1 $P_aO_2 \text{ (supine)} = 103.5 - (0.42 \times \text{Age})$

EQUATION 2 $P_aO_2 \text{ (seated)} = 104.2 - (0.27 \times \text{age})$

P_aO_2 (supine) :   Predicted P_aO_2 (mm Hg) in a supine position

P_aO_2 (seated) :   Predicted P_aO_2 (mm Hg) in a seated position

Age   :   Patient's age in years

EXAMPLE   What is the predicted P_aO_2 of a 60-year-old patient who is breathing spontaneously in a supine position?

$$
\begin{aligned}
P_aO_2 \text{ (supine)} &= 103.5 - (0.42 \times \text{age}) \\
&= 103.5 - (0.42 \times 60) \\
&= 103.5 - 25.2 \\
&= 78.3 \text{ or } 78 \text{ mm Hg}
\end{aligned}
$$

EXERCISE   Calculate the predicted P_aO_2 for a healthy 40-year-old patient who is spontaneously breathing room air in a sitting position.

[Answer: P_aO_2 (seated) = 93.4 or 93 mm Hg]

REFERENCES   Krider; Sorbini

SEE F_IO_2 Needed for a Desired P_aO_2.

SELF-ASSESSMENT QUESTIONS

67a. Given the equation to calculate the predicted PO_2 in a supine position: PO_2 (supine) = 103.5 − (0.42 × age). What is the predicted PO_2 of a 50-year-old patient who is breathing spontaneously in a supine position?

(A) 73 mm Hg
(B) 78 mm Hg
(C) 83 mm Hg
(D) 87 mm Hg

67b. Use the equation below to calculate the predicted PO_2 for a 50-year-old patient who is breathing room air spontaneously in a sitting position.

$$PO_2 \text{ (seated)} = 104.2 - (0.27 \times \text{age})$$

(A) 71 mm Hg
(B) 77 mm Hg
(C) 80 mm Hg
(D) 91 mm Hg

67c. Based on the study by Sorbini, the predicted P_aO_2 in healthy subjects decreases by _____ per year of age.

(A) 0.22 mm Hg
(B) 0.43 mm Hg
(C) 0.68 mm Hg
(D) 0.85 mm Hg

Chapter

68

Pressure Support Ventilation Setting

NOTES

To calculate the PSV setting, the $\dot{V}_{mach}$ and $\dot{V}_{spon}$ should have the same units of measurement (L/min or mL/sec).

Pressure support ventilation is used to reduce the work of spontaneous breathing by overcoming the airflow resistance during mechanical ventilation. PSV is active only when spontaneous breathing is available during mechanical ventilation (e.g., SIMV).

During *mechanical ventilation* and in patients with measurable spontaneous breathing efforts, the calculated PSV setting is used to overcome airflow resistance imposed by the endotracheal tube, secretions, and ventilator circuit. The calculated PSV setting is used during the initial phase of PSV. The PSV setting is adjusted based on the changing airflow resistance.

For *weaning* from mechanical ventilation using a *spontaneous breathing trial*, PSV is titrated until a spontaneous frequency of 20 to 25/min or a spontaneous tidal volume of 8 to 10 mL/kg ideal body weight (IBW) results. A PSV of greater than 30 cm H_2O is rarely needed as these patients are typically not ready for weaning. The PSV level is reduced by 2 to 4 cm H_2O increments as tolerated. Extubation can be considered when the PSV level reaches 5 to 8 cm H_2O for two hours with no signs of respiratory distress.

EQUATION

PSV setting = $[(\text{PIP} - P_{plat})/\dot{V}_{mach}] \times \dot{V}_{spon}$

PSV setting: Initial pressure support ventilation setting

PIP   :   Peak inspiratory pressure

P_{plat} :   Plateau pressure

$\dot{V}_{vent}$:   Inspiratory flow of ventilator, in L/min

$\dot{V}_{spon}$:   Inspiratory flow during spontaneous breathing in L/min (obtained via flow/time graphic *or* estimated to be 500 mL/sec or 30 L/min)

EXAMPLE

Calculate the PSV setting for a mechanically ventilated patient with the following data: PIP = 50 cm H_2O, P_{plat} = 35 cm H_2O, $\dot{V}_{vent}$ = 50 L/min, $\dot{V}_{spon}$ = 30 L/min).

$$\text{PSV setting} = \left[\frac{(\text{PIP} - P_{plat})}{\dot{V}_{mach}}\right] \times \dot{V}_{spon}$$

$$= \left[\frac{(50 \text{ cm } H_2O - 35 \text{ cm } H_2O)}{50 \text{ L/min}}\right] \times 30 \text{ L/min}$$

$$= \left[\frac{(15 \text{ cm } H_2O)}{50 \text{ L/min}}\right] \times 30 \text{ L/min}$$

$$= \left[\frac{(0.3 \text{ cm } H_2O)}{\text{L/min}}\right] \times 30 \text{ L/min}$$

$$= 9 \text{ cm } H_2O$$

The initial setting for pressure support ventilation is 9 cm H_2O.

EXERCISE 1

A mechanically ventilated patient has the following data: PIP = 45 cm H_2O, P_{plat} = 25 cm H_2O, $\dot{V}_{vent}$ = 60 L/min, $\dot{V}_{spon}$ = 30 L/min. Calculate the initial PSV setting.

[Answer: PSV setting = 10 cm H_2O]

EXERCISE 2

The following data are obtained from a patient who is being mechanically ventilated on a SIMV mode: PIP = 50 cm H_2O, P_{plat} = 35 cm H_2O, $\dot{V}_{vent}$ = 40 L/min, $\dot{V}_{spon}$ = 20 L/min. What should be the initial PSV setting.

[Answer: PSV setting = 7.5 cm H_2O]

REFERENCE   Wilkins (2)

chestjournal.chestpubs.org/content/93/4/795.full.pdf

SELF-ASSESSMENT QUESTIONS

68a. A patient is being mechanically ventilated, and the data below are obtained: PIP = 60 cm H_2O, P_{plat} = 40 cm H_2O, $\dot{V}_{vent}$ = 50 L/min, $\dot{V}_{spon}$ = 20 L/min. What should be the initial PSV setting?

(A) 6 cm H_2O
(B) 8 cm H_2O
(C) 10 cm H_2O
(D) 12 cm H_2O

$$\frac{60-40}{50} \times 20 \rightarrow \frac{20}{50} \times 20$$

$$0.4 \times 20 = 8 cm H_2O$$

68b. A respiratory therapist has recorded the following data from a mechanically ventilated patient: PIP = 50 cm H_2O, P_{plat} = 40 cm H_2O, $\dot{V}_{vent}$ = 60 L/min, $\dot{V}_{spon}$ = 30 L/min. Calculate the initial PSV setting.

(A) 5 cm H_2O
(B) 7 cm H_2O
(C) 9 cm H_2O
(D) 11 cm H_2O

$$\frac{50-40}{60} \times 30 \qquad \frac{10}{60} \times 30$$

$$0.167 \times 30 = 5 cm H_2O$$

68c. Pressure support ventilation *cannot* be used during which mode of ventilation?

(A) SIMV
(B) CMV
(C) CPAP
(D) IMV

68d. When weaning a patient from mechanical ventilation using a spontaneous breathing trial, the initial PSV level is titrated until a _____ is reached.

(A) spontaneous frequency of 25 to 30/min
(B) spontaneous tidal volume of 4 to 6 mL/kg IBW
(C) spontaneous frequency of 20 to 25/min
(D) spontaneous tidal volume of 6 to 8 mL/kg IBW

68e. The physician asks a therapist to perform a spontaneous breathing trial for weaning purpose. The respiratory therapist should titrate the PSV setting until the patient achieves a:

(A) spontaneous tidal volume of 6 mL/kg IBW
(B) spontaneous frequency of 30/min.
(C) spontaneous frequency of 12/min.
(D) spontaneous tidal volume of 10 mL/kg IBW

69

Relative Humidity

Relative humidity is usually measured by hygrometers, thus eliminating the need for extracting and measuring the humidity content of the air samples. The Examples illustrate how humidity content and capacity are related to the relative humidity.

Because the capacity is directly related to the temperature, a higher temperature causes the capacity to increase. If the content remains constant, a higher temperature or capacity ensures a *lower* relative humidity; the converse is also true.

Heated aerosol therapy provides two components to respiratory care. First, the heat increases the capacity of the gas mixture to carry humidity. Second, the aerosol increases the content (actual humidity) of the inspired gas, thus lowering the humidity deficit.

EQUATION

$$RH = \frac{Content}{Capacity}$$

RH : Relative humidity in %

Content : Humidity content of a volume of gas in mg/L or mm Hg; also known as actual or absolute humidity

Capacity : Humidity capacity or maximum amount of water that air can hold at a given temperature, in mg/L or mm Hg; also known as maximum absolute humidity.

NORMAL VALUE

The relative humidity is directly proportional to the content.

EXAMPLE 1

What is the relative humidity if the content of an air sample is 12 mg/L and its capacity is 18 mg/L?

$$RH = \frac{Content}{Capacity}$$
$$= \frac{12}{18}$$
$$= 0.67 \text{ or } 67\%$$

EXAMPLE 2

Calculate the relative humidity if the content of an air sample is 16 mg/L and its capacity is 18 mg/L.

$$RH = \frac{Content}{Capacity}$$
$$= \frac{16}{18}$$
$$= 0.89 \text{ or } 89\%$$

EXAMPLE 2

Calculate the relative humidity if the content of an air sample is 16 mg/L and its capacity is 20 mg/L.

$$RH = \frac{Content}{Capacity}$$
$$= \frac{16}{20}$$
$$= 0.8 \text{ or } 80\%$$

EXERCISE 1   An air sample has a humidity content of 15 mg/L and a capacity of 26 mg/L. What is the calculated relative humidity of this air sample?

[Answer: RH = 0.577 or 58%]

EXERCISE 2   Calculate the relative humidity of an air sample if the humidity content and capacity are 25 mg/L and 43 mg/L, respectively.

[Answer: RH = 0.581 or 58%]

REFERENCES   White; Wilkins (2)

SEE   *Humidity Deficit; Appendix F: Conversion Factors from ATPS to BTPS; Appendix R: Humidity Capacity of Saturated Gas at Selected Temperatures.*

SELF-ASSESSMENT QUESTIONS

69a. What is the relative humidity if the humidity content of an air sample is 12 mg/L and the humidity capacity is 24 mg/L?

(A) 20%
(B) 40%
(C) 50%
(D) 60%

69b. Calculate the relative humidity of an air sample if its humidity content is 14 mg/L and the humidity capacity is 19 mg/L.

(A) 33%
(B) 74%
(C) 80%
(D) 85%

69c. An air sample has a humidity content of 23 mg/L and a capacity of 26 mg/L at 100% saturation. Calculate the relative humidity of this sample.

(A) 32%
(B) 64%
(C) 78%
(D) 88%

Chapter

70

Reynolds' Number

NOTE

Osborne Reynolds (1842–1912), an English scientist, developed a dimensionless number (ratio) to describe the dynamics of fluid and air flows.

EQUATION

$$R_N = \frac{v \times D \times d}{\mu}$$

R_N : Reynolds number
v : Velocity of fluid
D : Fluid density
d : Diameter of tube
μ : Viscosity of fluid

When the Reynolds number is less than 2,000, it reflects laminar flow; when over 2,000, it reflects turbulent flow. In actuality, values between 2,000 and 4,000 provide a mixed or transitional pattern (laminar and turbulent), but most respiratory care references refer to values within this range as turbulent flow. The gas flow characteristics of this equation can be applied to respiratory care. An increase in gas flow rate (v) or gas density (D) will increase the Reynolds number, thus making a turbulent flow more likely. An oxygen/helium mixture has been used to reduce the gas density to enhance gas flow and diffusion of oxygen.

An increase in airway size (d) does not increase the Reynolds number because the resulting lower flow rate (v) resulting from larger airway diameter tends to offset any significant change in the Reynolds number.

REFERENCES   Barnes; Pierson; Wilkins (2); Wojciechowski

SELF-ASSESSMENT QUESTIONS

70a. Reynolds' number is used to describe the characteristic of:

(A) fluid and air flow.
(B) gas density.
(C) lung elasticity.
(D) lung compliance.

70b. Laminar flow is expected when the:

(A) flow is greater than 4 L/min
(B) flow is less than 4 L/min
(C) Reynolds' number is greater than 4,000.
(D) Reynolds' number is less than 2,000.

70c. Oxygen/helium mixtures have been used on patients with airway obstruction because these mixtures provide a(n) _____ of gas density and _____ gas flow and diffusion of oxygen.

(A) increase; increase
(B) decrease; decrease
(C) increase; decrease
(D) decrease; increase

70d. An increase in airway size _____ the Reynolds number because the resulting _____ flow rate ($\dot{V}$) offsets any significant change in Reynolds' number.

(A) increases; higher
(B) decreases; higher
(C) does not change; lower
(D) does not change; higher

Chapter

71

Shunt Equation ($Q_{sp}/\dot{Q}_T$): Classic Physiologic

NOTES

The shunt equation is used to calculate the portion of cardiac output not taking part in gas exchange-wasted perfusion. The classic physiologic shunt equation requires an arterial sample for C_aO_2 and a mixed venous sample for $C_{\bar{v}}O_2$.

A calculated shunt of less than 10% is considered normal in clinical settings. A shunt of 10 to 20% indicates mild intrapulmonary shunting, and a shunt of 20 to 30% indicates significant intrapulmonary shunting. Greater than 30% of calculated shunt reflects critical and severe intrapulmonary shunting. $Q_{sp}/\dot{Q}_T$ is increased in the presence of one of the following categories of shunt-producing diseases: *anatomic shunt* (e.g., congenital heart disease, intrapulmonary fistulas, vascular lung tumors); *capillary shunt* (e.g., atelectasis, alveolar fluid); *venous admixture* (e.g., hypoventilation, uneven distribution of ventilation, diffusion defects).

EQUATION

$$\frac{Q_{sp}}{\dot{Q}_T} = \frac{C_cO_2 - C_aO_2}{C_cO_2 - C_{\bar{v}}O_2}$$

$Q_{sp}/\dot{Q}_T$: Physiologic shunt to total perfusion ratio in %
C_cO_2 : End-capillary oxygen content in vol%
C_aO_2 : Arterial oxygen content in vol%
$C_{\bar{v}}O_2$: Mixed venous oxygen content in vol%

NORMAL VALUE

Less than 10%

EXAMPLE

Given: C_cO_2 = 20.4 vol%
C_aO_2 = 19.8 vol%
$C_{\bar{v}}O_2$ = 13.4 vol%

$$Q_{sp}/\dot{Q}_T = \frac{C_cO_2 - C_aO_2}{C_cO_2 - C_{\bar{v}}O_2}$$

$$= \frac{20.4 - 19.8}{20.4 - 13.4}$$

$$= \frac{0.6}{7}$$

$$= 0.086 \text{ or } 8.6\%$$

EXERCISE

Given: C_cO_2 = 20.6 vol%
C_aO_2 = 17.2 vol%
$C_{\bar{v}}O_2$ = 10.6 vol%

Calculate the $Q_{sp}/\dot{Q}_T$. Is it normal or abnormal?

[Answer: $Q_{sp}/\dot{Q}_T$ = 34%. Severe intrapulmonary shunting.]

REFERENCES

Malley; Shapiro

SEE

Oxygen Content: End-capillary (C_cO_2) for calculation of C_cO_2. Shunt Equation ($Q_{sp}/\dot{Q}_T$): Estimated; Appendix V: Oxygen Transport Normal Ranges.

SELF-ASSESSMENT QUESTIONS

71a. Normal cardiopulmonary function usually provides a calculated shunt of:

(A) 10% or less.
(B) 20% or less.
(C) 30% or less.
(D) 40% or less.

71b. The classic physiologic shunt equation is represented by:

(A) $(C_aO_2 - C_{\bar{v}}O_2) \times (C_cO_2 - C_aO_2)$

(B) $\dfrac{C_aO_2 - C_{\bar{v}}O_2}{C_cO_2 - C_aO_2}$

(C) $\dfrac{C_aO_2 - C_{\bar{v}}O_2}{C_cO_2 - C_aO_2}$

(D) $\dfrac{C_cO_2 - C_aO_2}{C_cO_2 - C_{\bar{v}}O_2}$

71c. The $(C_cO_2 - C_aO_2)$ portion of the classic physiologic shunt equation represents:

(A) oxygen consumption.
(B) shunted perfusion.
(C) total perfusion.
(D) oxygen content.

71d. Given: $C_cO_2 = 21.1$ vol%, $C_aO_2 = 18.8$ vol%, $C_{\bar{v}}O_2 = 14.4$ vol%. Calculate the percent shunt using the classic physiologic shunt equation. Is it normal or abnormal?

(A) 10%; normal
(B) 34%; abnormal
(C) 34%; normal
(D) 66%; abnormal

71e. Given: $C_cO_2 = 20.5$ vol%, $C_aO_2 = 20.1$ vol%, $C_{\bar{v}}O_2 = 13.8$ vol%. Calculate the percent shunt using the classic physiologic shunt equation. Is it normal or abnormal?

(A) 6%; normal
(B) 6%; abnormal
(C) 12%; normal
(D) 12%; abnormal

71f. A patient in the intensive care unit has the following oxygen content measurements: $C_aO_2 = 19.7$ vol%, $C_{\bar{v}}O_2 = 13.6$ vol%. If the calculated C_cO_2 is 20.8 vol%, what is the percent shunt based on the classic physiologic shunt equation? Is the calculated shunt normal, mild, moderate, or severe for this patient?

(A) 10%; normal shunt
(B) 10%; mild shunt
(C) 15%; mild shunt
(D) 15%; moderate shunt

71g. A patient who is diagnosed with adult respiratory distress syndrome has a C_cO_2 of 21 vol%, C_aO_2 of 18.2 vol%, and $C_{\bar{v}}O_2$ of 14 vol%. Use the classic physiologic shunt equation to calculate the shunt percent. Is it consistent with the diagnosis?

(A) 20%; mild shunt, inconsistent with diagnosis

(B) 30%; mild shunt, inconsistent with diagnosis

(C) 40%; moderate shunt, consistent with diagnosis

(D) 40%; severe shunt, consistent with diagnosis

71h. Which of the following sets of oxygen content measurement has the *highest* calculated physiologic shunt?

	C_cO_2	C_aO_2	$C_{\bar{v}}O_2$ (vol%)
(A)	20	19	15
(B)	19	17	14
(C)	21	20	16
(D)	18	17	13

71i. Which of the following sets of oxygen content measurement has the *lowest* calculated physiologic shunt?

	C_cO_2	C_aO_2	$C_{\bar{v}}O_2$ (vol%)
(A)	20.8	18.7	14.3
(B)	18.7	16.9	13.2
(C)	20.1	19.0	14.6
(D)	18.4	17.2	13.5

71j. Which of the following sets of oxygen content measurement represents *normal* physiologic shunt?

	C_cO_2	C_aO_2	$C_{\bar{v}}O_2$ (vol%)
(A)	19.8	19.0	14.3
(B)	20.3	18.2	13.6
(C)	17.1	16.8	12.9
(D)	18.3	17.5	13.8

71k. A patient has a series of physiologic shunts measured; they are listed as follows. Which of the following sets of oxygen content measurements represents a severe physiologic shunt?

	C_cO_2	C_aO_2	$C_{\bar{v}}O_2$ (vol%)
(A)	20.3	17.8	13.6
(B)	19.6	19.0	14.7
(C)	19.1	17.7	13.5
(D)	18.5	17.9	13.8

Chapter

72

Shunt Equation ($Q_{sp}/\dot{Q}_T$): Estimated

NOTES

The estimated shunt equation does not require a mixed venous blood sample. It is less accurate than the classic physiologic shunt equation. In normal subjects, 5 vol% may be used as the estimated arterial-mixed venous oxygen content difference $\{C(a-\bar{v})O_2\}$. In critically ill patients, 3.5 vol% may be used as it is common for these patients to have a lower $C(a-\bar{v})O_2$ as a result of increased cardiac output or decreased oxygen consumption (extraction).

A calculated shunt of less than 10% is considered normal in clinical settings. A shunt of 10 to 20% indicates mild intrapulmonary shunting, and a shunt of 20 to 30% is indicative of significant intrapulmonary shunting. Greater than 30% of calculated shunt reflects critical and severe intrapulmonary shunting.

$Q_{sp}/\dot{Q}_T$ is increased in the presence of one of the following categories of shunt-producing disease: *anatomic shunt* (e.g., congenital heart disease, intrapulmonary fistulas, vascular lung tumors); *capillary shunt* (e.g., atelectasis, alveolar fluid); *venous admixture* (e.g., hypoventilation, uneven distribution of ventilation, diffusion defects).

EQUATION 1

For individuals who are breathing spontaneously with or without CPAP:

$$\frac{Q_{sp}}{\dot{Q}_T} = \frac{C_cO_2 - C_aO_2}{5 + (C_cO_2 - C_aO_2)}$$

EQUATION 2

For critically ill patients who are receiving mechanical ventilation with or without *PEEP*:

$$\frac{Q_{sp}}{\dot{Q}_T} = \frac{C_cO_2 - C_aO_2}{3.5 + (C_cO_2 - C_aO_2)}$$

$Q_{sp}/\dot{Q}_T$: Physiologic shunt to total perfusion ration in %
C_cO_2 : End-capillary oxygen content in vol%
C_aO_2 : Arterial oxygen content in vol%

NORMAL VALUE

Less than 10%

EXAMPLE 1

Given: A patient on CPAP of 5 cm H_2O
C_cO_2 = 20.4 vol%
C_aO_2 = 19.8 vol%
Use 5 vol% as the estimated $C(a-\bar{v})O_2$ and calculate $Q_{sp}/\dot{Q}_T$.

$$\frac{Q_{sp}}{\dot{Q}_T} = \frac{C_cO_2 - C_aO_2}{5 + (C_cO_2 - C_aO_2)}$$

$$= \frac{20.4 - 19.8}{5 + (20.4 - 19.8)}$$

$$= \frac{0.6}{5 + 0.6}$$

$$= \frac{0.6}{5.6}$$

$$= 0.107 \text{ or } 10.7\%$$

EXAMPLE 2

Given: A patient on mechanical ventilation

$C_cO_2 = 20.4$ vol%

$C_aO_2 = 19.8$ vol%

Use 3.5 vol% as the estimated $C(a-\bar{v})O_2$ and calculate $Q_{sp}/\dot{Q}_T$.

$$\frac{Q_{sp}}{\dot{Q}_T} = \frac{C_cO_2 - C_aO_2}{3.5 + (C_cO_2 - C_aO_2)}$$

$$= \frac{20.4 - 19.8}{3.5 + (20.4 - 19.8)}$$

$$= \frac{0.6}{3.5 + 0.6}$$

$$= \frac{0.6}{4.1}$$

$$= 0.146 \text{ or } 14.6\%$$

EXERCISE 1

Given: $C_cO_2 = 20.6$ vol%

$\quad\quad\quad C_aO_2 = 19.8$ vol%

Use $C(a-\bar{v})O_2$ of 5 vol% and calculate the estimated $Q_{sp}/\dot{Q}_T$ of a patient. Is it normal?

[Answer: $Q_{sp}/\dot{Q}_T = 0.138$ or 13.8%. Abnormal, mild shunt.]

EXERCISE 2

Given the oxygen contents of a critically ill patient who is receiving mechanical ventilation:

$C_cO_2 = 20.6$ vol%

$C_aO_2 = 17.2$ vol%

Use $C(a-\bar{v})O_2$ of 3.5 vol% and calculate the estimated $Q_{sp}/\dot{Q}_T$ of this critically ill patient. Is it normal?

[Answer: $Q_{sp}/\dot{Q}_T = 0.49$ or 4.9%. Abnormal, severe shunt.]

REFERENCES

Malley; Shapiro

SEE

Shunt Equation $Q_{sp}/\dot{Q}_T$: Classic Physiologic; Appendix V: Oxygen Transport.

SELF-ASSESSMENT QUESTIONS

72a. All of the following are true with regard to the estimated shunt equation with the *exception* of:

(A) it does not require placement of a pulmonary artery catheter.

(B) it does not require a mixed venous sample.

(C) its accuracy is the same as the classic physiologic shunt equation.

(D) it requires only an arterial blood sample.

72b. Select the estimated physiologic shunt equation for individuals who are not receiving mechanical ventilation:

(A) $\dfrac{C_cO_2 - C_aO_2}{C_cO_2 - C_{\bar{v}}O_2}$

(B) $(C_cO_2 - C_aO_2) \times (5 + C_cO_2 - C_aO_2)$

(C) $\dfrac{C_cO_2 - C_aO_2}{5 + C_cO_2 - C_aO_2}$

(D) $\dfrac{C_aO_2 - C_{\bar{v}}O_2}{5 + C_cO_2 - C_aO_2}$

72c. Given: $C_cO_2 = 20.4$ vol%, $C_aO_2 = 19.7$ vol%. Calculate the estimated $\dfrac{Q_{SP}}{\dot{Q}_T}$. Is it normal? (Assume $C_aO_2 - C_{\bar{v}}O_2 = 5$ vol% for individuals not receiving mechanical ventilation).

(A) 12.3%; normal
(B) 12.3%; mild shunt
(C) 23.6%; normal
(D) 23.6%; moderate shunt

72d. A *critically ill* patient has a C_aO_2 of 14.5 vol%. If the calculated end-capillary oxygen content is 16.8 vol%, what is the estimated shunt for this patient? How severe is the shunt? (Assume $C_aO_2 - C_{\bar{v}}O_2 = 3.5$ vol% for critically ill patients.)

(A) 24.8%; mild shunt
(B) 24.8%; moderate shunt
(C) 39.6%; moderate shunt
(D) 39.6%; severe shunt

72e. Which of the following sets of values has the *highest* estimated shunt?

	C_cO_2	C_aO_2 (vol%)
(A)	20	19
(B)	19	17
(C)	21	20
(D)	18	17

72f. Which of the following sets of values has the *lowest* estimated shunt?

	C_cO_2	C_aO_2 (vol%)
(A)	20.8	18.7
(B)	18.7	16.9
(C)	20.1	19.0
(D)	18.4	17.2

72g. Which of the following sets of values represents a *normal* estimated shunt?

	C_cO_2	C_aO_2 (vol%)
(A)	19.8	19.0
(B)	20.3	18.2
(C)	17.1	16.8
(D)	18.3	17.5

72h. A patient's arterial oxygen contents are shown below. With the respective end-capillary oxygen content, which of the following sets of values shows a severe physiologic shunt?

	C_cO_2	C_aO_2 (vol%)
(A)	20.3	17.8
(B)	19.6	19.0
(C)	19.1	17.7
(D)	18.5	17.9

72i. The following values are obtained from a *critically ill* patient: $C_cO_2 = 20.5$ vol%, $C_aO_2 = 18.6$ vol%, $C_{\bar{v}}O_2 = 14.8$ vol%. Calculate the percent shunt using the classic physiologic shunt equation. Assuming $C_aO_2 - C_{\bar{v}}O_2 = 3.5$ vol%, calculate the estimated shunt.

(A) classic 33.3%; estimated 35.2%
(B) classic 33.3%; estimated 36.5%
(C) classic 34.1%; estimated 27.5%
(D) classic 34.1%; estimated 36.5%

Chapter

73

Shunt Equation: Modified

EQUATION

$$\frac{Qs}{\dot{Q}_T} = \frac{(P_A O2 - P_a O_2) \times 0.003}{(C_a O_2 - C_{\bar{v}} O_2) + (P_A O_2 - P_a O_2) \times 0.003}$$

$\dfrac{Qs}{\dot{Q}_T}$: Modified shunt in %

$P_A O_2$: Alveolar oxygen tension in mm Hg
$P_a O_2$: Arterial oxygen tension in mm Hg
$C_a O_2$: Arterial oxygen content in vol%
$C_{\bar{v}} O_2$: Mixed venous oxygen content in vol%

This equation is modified from the classic physiologic shunt equation in which $(P_A O_2 - P_a O_2) \times 0.003$ is used to substitute for $C_c O_2 - C_a O_2$. The equation requires an arterial PO_2 greater than 150 mm Hg. As most patients do not achieve this level of PO_2, it has limited clinical application.

A further simplified equation, $P_A O_2 - P_a O_2$, consisting of only a portion of the modified shunt equation, has been used to estimate the degree of physiologic shunt. To increase the accuracy of this simplified equation, the $P_A O_2$ and $P_a O_2$ values are usually measured on an $F_I O_2$ of 100%.

REFERENCE

Barnes

SEE

Shunt Equation: Classic Physiologic, Alveolar–Arterial Oxygen Tension Gradient P(A−a)O₂.

SELF-ASSESSMENT QUESTIONS

73a. In the modified shunt equation, $(P_A O_2 - P_a O_2) \times 0.003$ is used to substitute for _____ of the classic physiologic shunt equation.

(A) $C_c O_2 - C_a O_2$
(B) $C_a O_2 - C_{\bar{v}} O_2$
(C) $C_{\bar{v}} O_2 - C_a O_2$
(D) $C_c O_2 - C_{\bar{v}} O_2$

73b. To be accurate, the modified shunt equation should have an arterial PO_2 greater than _____ mm Hg.

(A) 100

(B) 120

(C) 150

(D) 200

73c. Which of the following statements is true in regard to the modified shunt equation?

(A) It does not require a mixed venous sample.

(B) It does not require a P_AO_2 value.

(C) It is the most commonly used shunt equation.

(D) It requires two blood gas samples.

Chapter

74

Stroke Volume (*SV*) and Stroke Volume Index (*SVI*)

NOTES

The stroke volume (*SV*) measures the average cardiac output per one heartbeat. Its accuracy is dependent on the method and technique used in the cardiac output measurement (e.g., Fick's estimated method, dye-dilution, and thermodilution).

The *SV* is increased by drugs that raise cardiac contractility and during early stages of compensated septic shock. It is decreased by drugs that lower cardiac contractility and during late stages of decompensated septic shock.

The stroke volume index (*SVI*) is used to normalize stroke volume measurement among patients of varying body size. For instance, a 50-mL stroke volume may be normal for an average-sized person but low for a large person. The *SVI* can distinguish this difference based on the body size. See Table 2-10 for factors that change *SV, SVI*, and other hemodynamic measurements.

EQUATION 1

$$SV = \frac{CO}{HR}$$

EQUATION 2

$$SVI = \frac{SV}{BSA}$$

SV : Stroke volume in mL or mL/beat
SVI : Stroke volume index in mL/m^2 (or mL/beat/m^2)
CO : Cardiac output in L/min ($\dot{Q}_T$)
HR : Heart rate/min
BSA : Body surface area in m^2

NORMAL VALUES

SV : 40 to 80 mL

SVI : 33 to 47 mL/m^2

EXAMPLE

Given: Cardiac output = 4.0 L/min
Heart rate = 100/min
Body surface area = 1.5 m^2

Calculate the stroke volume and the stroke volume index.

$$SV = \frac{CO}{HR}$$

$$= \frac{4.0}{100}$$

$$= 0.04 \text{ L or } 40 \text{ mL}$$

$$SVI = \frac{SV}{BSA}$$

$$= \frac{40}{1.5}$$

$$= 26.7 \text{ mL/m}^2$$

TABLE 2-10 Factors Increasing and Decreasing Stroke Volume (*SV*), Stroke Volume Index (*SVI*), Cardiac Output (*CO*), Cardiac Index (*CI*), Right Ventricular Stroke Work Index (*RVSWI*), and Left Ventricular Stroke Work Index (*LVSWI*)

INCREASES	DECREASES
Positive Inotrophic Drugs (Increased Contractility)	**Negative Inotropic Drugs (Decreased Contractility)**
Dobutamine (Dobutrex®)	Propranolol (Inderal®)
Epinephrine (Adrenalin®)	Timolol (Blocadren®)
Dopamine (Intropin®)	Metoprolol (Lopressor®)
Isoproterenol (Isuprel®)	Atenolol (Tenormin®)
Digitalis	Nadolol (Corgard®)
Amrinone (Inocor®)	
Abnormal Conditions	**Abnormal Conditions**
Septic shock (early stages)	Septic shock (later stages)
Hyperthermia	Congestive heart failure
Hypervolemia	Hypovolemia
Decreased vascular resistance	Pulmonary emboli
	Increased vascular resistance
	Myocardial infarction
	Hyperinflation of Lungs
	Mechanical ventilation
	Positive End-Expiratory Pressure (*PEEP*)

EXERCISE

Given: Cardiac output = 5.0 L/min
Heart rate = 80/min
Body surface area = 1.2 m^2
Calculate the stroke volume and the stroke volume index.

[Answer: $SV = 62.5$ mL; $SVI = 52.1$ mL/m^2]

REFERENCE

Des Jardins

SEE

Cardiac Output CO: Fick's Estimated Method; Cardiac Index (CI); Appendix I: DuBois Body Surface Chart; Appendix Q: Hemodynamic Normal Ranges.

SELF-ASSESSMENT QUESTIONS

74a. The equation for calculating the stroke volume (*SV*) is:

(A) Cardiac output $\times$ Heart rate

(B) $\dfrac{\text{Cardiac output}}{\text{Heart rate}}$

(C) $\dfrac{\text{Cardiac output} \times \text{Heart rate}}{\text{Body surface area}}$

(D) $\dfrac{\text{Cardiac output / Heart rate}}{\text{Body surface area}}$

74b. The equation for calculating the stroke volume index (*SVI*) is:

(A) Cardiac output $\times$ Heart rate

(B) $\dfrac{\text{Cardiac output}}{\text{Heart rate}}$

(C) $\dfrac{\text{Cardiac output} \times \text{Heart rate}}{\text{Body surface area}}$

(D) $\dfrac{\text{Cardiac output / Heart rate}}{\text{Body surface area}}$

74c. Given: cardiac output = 4.5 L/min. heart rate = 110/min. body surface area = 1.3 m^2. Calculate the stroke volume (*SV*) and stroke volume index (*SVI*).

(A) $SV = 46.2$ mL; $SVI = 35.5$ mL/m^2

(B) $SV = 44.6$ mL; $SVI = 34.3$ mL/m^2

(C) $SV = 42.0$ mL; $SVI = 32.3$ mL/m^2

(D) $SV = 40.9$ mL; $SVI = 31.5$ mL/m^2

Handwritten: 4.5L/min / 110min = 0.0409 = 40.9mL; 40.9 ÷ 1.3m² = 31.46

74d. A patient whose body surface area is about 1.1 m^2 has the following hemodynamic measurements: cardiac output = 5.9 L/min, heart rate = 120/min. Calculate the stroke volume (*SV*) and stroke volume index (*SVI*).

(A) $SV = 70.8$ mL; $SVI = 51.6$ mL/m^2

(B) $SV = 70.8$ mL; $SVI = 64.4$ mL/m^2

(C) $SV = 49.2$ mL; $SVI = 40.7$ mL/m^2

(D) $SV = 49.2$ mL; $SVI = 44.7$ mL/m^2

Handwritten: 5.9/120 = 49.2; 49.2/1.1m² = 44.69 = 44.7

74e. Given the following stroke volume (*SV*) and body surface area (*BSA*) measurements, which set of values has the highest stroke volume index (*SVI*)?

	SV (mL)	*BSA* (m^2)	
(A)	60	1.4	*42.9*
(B)	55	1.2	*45.8*
(C)	58	2.0	*29.0*
(D)	63	1.7	*37.06*

75

Stroke Work: Left Ventricular (*LVSW*) and Index (*LVSWI*)

NOTES

Left ventricular stroke work (*LVSW*) reflects the work of the left heart in providing perfusion through the systemic circulation. *LVSW* is directly related to the systemic vascular resistance, myocardial mass, and the volume and viscosity of the blood. In addition, tachycardia, hypoxemia, and poor contractility of the heart may further increase the stroke work of the left heart.

The pulmonary capillary wedge pressure (*PCWP*) is used because it approximates the mean left atrial pressure or the left ventricle end-diastolic pressure.

The constant 0.0136 in the equation is used to convert mm Hg/mL to gram · meters (g · m).

The left ventricular stroke work index (*LVSWI*) is used to equalize the stroke work to a person's body size. In the example shown, an apparently low left ventricular stroke work may be normal for a small person after indexing. See Figure 2-39 for the relationship between *LVSWI* and left ventricular preload (represented by *PCWP*). For example, when the *LVSWI* and *PCWP* readings are both low and meet in quadrant 1, hypovolemia may be present.

EQUATION 1

$$LVSW = (MAP - PCWP) \times SV \times 0.0136$$

EQUATION 2

$$LVSWI = \frac{LVSW}{BSA}$$

LVSW : Left ventricular stroke work in g · m/beat
LVSWI : Left ventricular stroke work index in g · m/beat/m^2
MAP : Mean arterial pressure in mm Hg
PCWP : Pulmonary capillary wedge pressure in mm Hg
SV : Stroke volume in mL
BSA : Body surface area in m^2

NORMAL VALUES

LVSW = 60 to 80 g · m/beat
LVSWI = 40 to 60 g · m/beat/m^2

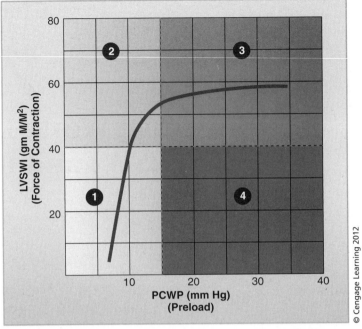

Figure 2-39 Frank-Starling curve. The Frank-Starling curve shows that the more the myocardial fiber is stretched as a result of the blood pressure that develops as blood returns to the chambers of the heart during diastole, the more the heart muscle contracts during systole. In addition, it contracts with greater force. The stretch produced within the myocardium at end-diastole is called preload. Clinically, it would be best to determine the preload of the left ventricle by measuring the end-diastolic pressure of the left ventricle or left atrium. However, because it is impractical to measure that at the patient's bedside, the best preload approximation of the left heart is the pulmonary capillary wedge pressure (PCWP). As shown in this illustration, the relationship of the PCWP (preload) to the left ventricular stroke work index (LVSWI) (force of contraction) may appear in four quadrants: (1) hypovolemia, (2) optimal function, (3) hypervolemia, and (4) cardiac failure.

EXAMPLE

Given: MAP = 100 mm Hg
$\quad\quad PCWP$ = 20 mm Hg
$\quad\quad SV$ = 50 mL
$\quad\quad BSA$ = 1.1 m^2

Calculate the left ventricular stroke work (*LVSW*) and its index (*LVSWI*).

$$LVSW = (\text{MAP} - \text{PCWP}) \times 50 \times 0.0136$$
$$= (100 - 20) \times 50 \times 0.0136$$
$$= 80 \times 50 \times 0.0136$$
$$= 4{,}000 \times 0.0136$$
$$= 54.4 \text{ g} \cdot \text{m/beat}$$
$$LVSWI = \frac{LVSW}{BSA}$$
$$= \frac{54.4}{1.1}$$
$$= 49.45 \text{ g} \cdot \text{m/beat/m}^2$$

EXERCISE

Given: MAP = 120 mm Hg
$\quad\quad PCWP$ = 20 mm Hg
$\quad\quad SV$ = 45 mL
$\quad\quad BSA$ = 1.5 m^2

Calculate the *LVSW* and *LVSWI*.

[Answer: *LVSW* = 61.2 g·m/beat; *LVSWI* = 40.8 g·m/beat/m²]

REFERENCE   Des Jardins

SEE   *Stroke Work: Right Ventricular (RVSW) and Index (RVSWI); Appendix Q: Hemodynamic Normal Ranges.*

SELF-ASSESSMENT QUESTIONS

75a. Calculation of the left ventricular stroke work (*LVSW*) and left ventricular stroke work index (*LVSWI*) does not require measurement of:

(A) mean arterial pressure.
(B) mean pulmonary arterial pressure.
(C) pulmonary capillary wedge pressure.
(D) stroke volume.

75b. The equation for calculating the left ventricular stroke work (*LVSW*) is:

(A) $(MAP + PCWP) \times SV.$
(B) $(MAP + PCWP) \times SV \times 0.0136.$
(C) $(MAP - PCWP) \times SV \times 0.0136.$
(D) $(MAP - PCWP) \times SV.$

75c. Given: *MAP* = 112 mm Hg, *PCWP* = 10 mm Hg, *SV* = 60 mL. What is the calculated left ventricular stroke work (*LVSW*)?

(A) 77.4 g · m/beat
(B) 80.1 g · m/beat
(C) 83.2 g · m/beat
(D) 89.7 g · m/beat

$(112 - 10) \times 60mL \times 0.0136$
$102 \times 60 = 6120 \times 0.0136 =$
$= 83.232$

75d. A patient whose estimated body surface area is 1.4 m² has the following hemodynamic values: *MAP* = 103 mm Hg, *PCWP* = 15 mm Hg, *SV* = 50 mL. What is the patient's left ventricular stroke work index (*LVSWI*)?

(A) 42.7 g · m/beat/m²
(B) 45.5 g · m/beat/m²
(C) 50.6 g · m/beat/m²
(D) 59.8 g · m/beat/m²

$(103 - 15) \times 50mL \times 0.0136$
$88 \times 50 = 4,400 = \dfrac{59.84}{BSA} = 42.7$

75e. The hemodynamic values for a patient (body surface area = 1.3 m²) in the coronary care unit are as follows: *MAP* = 133 mm Hg, *CVP* = 4 mm Hg, *PAP* = 28 mm Hg, *PCWP* = 15 mm Hg, *SV* = 55 mL. What is the patient's left ventricular stroke work (*LVSW*) and index (*LVSWI*)?

(A) *LVSW* = 79.5 g · m/beat; *LVSWI* = 61.1 g · m/beat/m²
(B) *LVSW* = 88.3 g · m/beat; *LVSWI* = 61.1 g · m/beat/m²
(C) *LVSW* = 88.3 g · m/beat; *LVSWI* = 67.9 g · m/beat/m²
(D) *LVSW* = 79.5 g · m/beat; *LVSWI* = 67.9 g · m/beat/m²

$(133 - 15) \times 55 \times 0.0136$
$118 \times 55 \times 0.0136 =$
88.264

Chapter

76

Stroke Work: Right Ventricular (*RVSW*) and Index (*RVSWI*)

Right ventricular stroke work (*RVSW*) reflects the work of the right heart in providing perfusion through the pulmonary circulation. *RVSW* is directly related to the pulmonary vascular resistance, myocardial mass, and the volume and viscosity of the blood. In addition, tachycardia, hypoxemia, and poor contractility of the heart may further increase the stroke work of the right heart.

The constant 0.0136 in the equation is used to convert mm Hg/mL to gram · meters (g · m).

The right ventricular stroke work index (*RVSWI*) is used to equalize the stroke work to a person's body size. In the example shown, an apparently normal *RVSW* may be low for a large person after indexing (normal *RVSW*, low *RVSWI*).

EQUATION 1

$$RVSW = (mPAP - \overline{RA}) \times SV \times 0.0136$$

EQUATION 2

$$RVSWI = \frac{RVSW}{BSA}$$

RVSW : Right ventricular stroke work in g · m/beat
RVSWI : Right ventricular stroke work index in g · m/beat/m^2
mPAP : Mean pulmonary artery pressure in mm Hg
$\overline{RA}$: Mean right atrial pressure in mm Hg
SV : Stroke volume in mL
BSA : Body surface area in m^2

NORMAL VALUES

$RVSW$ = 10 to 15 g · m/beat
$RVSWI$ = 7 to 12 g · m/beat/m^2

EXAMPLE

Given: $mPAP$ = 18 mm Hg
$\overline{RA}$ = 4 mm Hg
SV = 60 mL
BSA = 1.9 m^2

Calculate the right ventricular stroke work (*RVSW*) and its index (*RVSWI*).

$$RVSW = \left(mPAP - \overline{RA}\right) \times SV \times 0.0136$$
$$= (18 - 4) \times 60 \times 0.0136$$
$$= 14 \times 60 \times 0.0136$$
$$= 840 \times 0.0136$$
$$= 11.42 \text{ g} \cdot \text{m/beat}$$

$$RVSWI = \frac{RVSW}{BSA}$$
$$= \frac{11.42}{1.9}$$
$$= 6.01 \text{ g} \cdot \text{m/beat/m}^2$$

EXERCISE

Given: $mPAP$ = 20 mm Hg
$\overline{RA}$ = 6 mm Hg
SV = 56 mL
BSA = 1.2 m^2

Calculate the *RVSW* and *RVSWI*.

[Answer: $RVSW$ = 10.66 g · m/beat; $RVSWI$ = 8.88 g · m/beat/m^2]

REFERENCE

Bustin

SEE

Stroke Work: Left Ventricular (LVSW) and Index (LVSWI); Appendix Q: Hemodynamic Normal Ranges.

SELF-ASSESSMENT QUESTIONS

76a. Which of the following is not required for calculating the right ventricular stroke work (*RVSW*) and right ventricular stroke work index (*RVSWI*)?

(A) 0.0136
(B) Mean pulmonary artery pressure
(C) Systemic artery pressure
(D) Body surface area

76b. The equation for calculating the right ventricular stroke work (*RVSW*) is:

(A) $(mPAP - \overline{RA}) \times SV.$
(B) $(mPAP + \overline{RA}) \times SV \times 0.0136.$
(C) $(mPAP + \overline{RA}) \times SV.$
(D) $(mPAP - \overline{RA}) \times SV \times 0.0136.$

76c. Given: $mPAP$ = 20 mm Hg, $\overline{RA}$ = 3 mm Hg, SV = 55 mL. What is the calculated right ventricular stroke work (*RVSW*)?

(A) 11.4 g · m/beat
(B) 12.7 g · m/beat
(C) 13.9 g · m/beat
(D) 15.2 g · m/beat

$= (20 \text{ mm Hg} - 3) \times 55 \text{ mL} \times 0.0136$

$17 \times 55 = 935 \times 0.0136$

$= 127.16 = 12.7$

76d. Given: $mPAP$ = 22 mm Hg, $\overline{RA}$ = 6 mm Hg, SV = 45 mL, BSA = 1.1 m^2. Calculate the right ventricular stroke work index (*RVSWI*).

(A) 8.9 g · m/beat/m^2
(B) 9.1 g · m/beat/m^2
(D) 9.3 g · m/beat/m^2
(D) 9.8 g · m/beat/m^2

$(22 - 6) \times 45 \times 0.0136$

$720 \times 0.0136 =$

$\dfrac{9.792}{1.1} = 8.90$

$18 - 3 \times 60 \times 0.0136 =$

12.24

———————

$1.2 \, m^2 =$

$\downarrow$

10.2

76e. A patient whose estimated body surface area is 1.2 m^2 has the following hemodynamic values: $mPAP$ = 18 mm Hg, $\overline{RA}$ = 3 mm Hg, SV = 60 mL. What is the patient's right ventricular stroke work ($RVSW$) and right ventricular stroke work index ($RVSWI$)?

(A) $RVSW$ = 9.8 g · m/beat; $RVSWI$ = 8.2 g · m/beat/m^2

(B) $RVSW$ = 10.3 g · m/beat; $RVSWI$ = 8.6 g · m/beat/m^2

(C) $RVSW$ = 11.6 g · m/beat; $RVSWI$ = 9.7 g · m/beat/m^2

(D) $RVSW$ = 12.2 g · m/beat; $RVSWI$ = 10.2 g · m/beat/m^2

76f. A patient in the intensive care unit whose body surface area is about 1.4 m^2 has the following hemodynamic values: $mPAP$ = 20 mm Hg; $\overline{RA}$ = 6 mm Hg, SV = 65 mL. What is the patient's right ventricular stroke work ($RVSW$) and index ($RVSWI$)? Is the index normal?

(A) $RVSW$ = 12.38 g · m/beat; $RVSWI$ = 9.2 g · m/beat/m^2; normal

(B) $RVSW$ = 12.38 g · m/beat; $RVSWI$ = 8.8 g · m/beat/m^2; abnormal

(C) $RVSW$ = 16.17 g · m/beat; $RVSWI$ = 9.2 g · m/beat/m^2; normal

(D) $RVSW$ = 16.17 g · m/beat; $RVSWI$ = 8.8 g · m/beat/m^2; abnormal

$(20 - 6) \times 65 \times 0.0136$

$= 12.38 \div 1.4 \, m^2 = 8.84$

Chapter

77

Temperature Conversion
(°C to °F)

NOTES

Temperature conversion calculations are often done in pulmonary function and blood gas laboratories where a conversion chart is not readily available. It is essential to memorize the equation. In the Example, conversion of normal body temperature (from 37°C to 98.6°F) was done. If you are unsure of the °C to °F temperature conversion equation, you may first use these two numbers to check for its accuracy.

The temperature constant $\frac{9}{5}$ can be substituted by 1.8 in Celsius to Fahrenheit conversions.

EQUATION

$$°F = \left[°C \times \frac{9}{5} \right] + 32$$

°F : degrees Fahrenheit
°C : degrees Celsius

EXAMPLE

Given: °C = 37
Calculate the degrees Fahrenheit.

$$°F = \left[°C \times \frac{9}{5} \right] + 32$$

$$= \left[37 \times \frac{9}{5} \right] + 32$$

$$= \left[\frac{333}{5} \right] + 32$$

$$= 66.6 + 32$$

$$= 98.6$$

EXERCISE 1

Given: °C = 25
Find the degrees Fahrenheit.

[Answer: °F = 77]

EXERCISE 2

Given: °C = 39
Find the degrees Fahrenheit.

[Answer: °F = 102.2]

REFERENCE

Wilkins (2)

SEE

Temperature Conversion (°F to °C).

SELF-ASSESSMENT QUESTIONS

77a. Given: °C = 25. Calculate the degrees Fahrenheit.

   (A) 70°F
   (B) 73°F
   (C) 77°F
   (D) 79°F

77b. What is the normal body temperature (37 °C) in degrees Fahrenheit?

   (A) 96.2°F
   (B) 97.3°F
   (C) 98.1°F
   (D) 98.6°F

77c. The skin temperature of a neonate is recorded as 36 °C. What is its equivalent in degrees Fahrenheit?

   (A) 96.8°F
   (B) 97.4°F
   (C) 98.3°F
   (D) 98.9°F

77d. The freezing point of water is 0 °C. In degrees Fahrenheit, it is the same as:

   (A) 0°F.
   (B) 21°F.
   (C) 32°F.
   (D) 100°F.

Chapter

78

Temperature Conversion (°C to K)

NOTES

In respiratory care, the Kelvin (K or T) temperature scale is primarily used in gas law calculations (i.e., Boyle's law, Charles' law, Gay-Lussac's law, and Combined Gas Law).

Kelvin temperature is also called the absolute temperature because molecular activity of gases theoretically stops at 0 K (−273°C). In the Equation, it is essential to remember the constant number 273.

For temperature conversion from Fahrenheit (°F) to kelvins (K), change °F to °C and then use the Equation to solve for K.

EQUATION

$K = °C + 273$
K : kelvins
°C : degrees Celsius

EXAMPLE

Given: °C = 37
Calculate the Kelvin equivalent.
$$K = °C + 273$$
$$= 37 + 273$$
$$= 310$$

EXERCISE 1

Given: °C = 25
Find the Kelvin equivalent.

[Answer: K = 298]

EXERCISE 2

Given: °C = 39
Find the Kelvin equivalent.

[Answer: K = 312]

REFERENCE

Wilkins (2)

SELF-ASSESSMENT QUESTIONS

78a. The equation to convert a known temperature to kelvins is:

(A) 273 − °C.
(B) °C + 273.
(C) 273 − °F.
(D) °F + 273.

78b. Given: °C = 25. Calculate the kelvin equivalent.

(A) 360
(B) 240
(C) 298
(D) 304

78c. Given: °F = 88 (31°C). Calculate the kelvin equivalent.

(A) 360

(B) 325

(C) 312

(D) 304

78d. A gas volume is measured at 26°C. Find its equivalent in kelvins (K) for temperature correction with the Combined Gas Law.

(A) 247 K

(B) 288 K

(C) 299 K

(D) 330 K

78e. Which of the following gas temperatures is the same as 310 K?

(A) 35°C

(B) 37°C

(C) 39°C

(D) 94°F

Chapter

79

Temperature Conversion
(°F to °C)

NOTES

NOTES

Temperature conversion calculations are often done in pulmonary function and blood gas laboratories where a conversion chart is not readily available. It is essential to memorize the equation. In the Example, conversion of normal body temperature (from 98.6°F to 37°C) was done. If you are unsure of the °F to °C temperature conversion equation, you may first use these two numbers to check for its accuracy.

To convert Fahrenheit to kelvins, first change Fahrenheit to Celsius and then change to kelvins.

EQUATION

$$^{\circ}C = \left(^{\circ}F - 32\right) \times \frac{5}{9}$$

°C : degrees Celsius
°F : degrees Fahrenheit

EXAMPLE

Given: °F = 98.6
Calculate the degrees Celsius.

$$^{\circ}C = (^{\circ}F - 32) \times \frac{5}{9}$$

$$= (98.6 - 32) \times \frac{5}{9}$$

$$= (66.6) \times \frac{5}{9}$$

$$= \frac{333}{9}$$

$$= 37$$

EXERCISE

Given: °F = 100
Find the degrees Celsius.

[Answer: °C = 37.77 or 37.8]

REFERENCE

Wilkins (2)

SEE

Temperature Conversion (°C to K); Temperature Conversion (°C to °F).

SELF-ASSESSMENT QUESTIONS

79a. A patient has an oral temperature of 99.2°F. It is the same as:

(A) 36.8°C.
(B) 37.3°C.
(C) 37.7°C.
(D) 38.1°C.

79b. The rectal temperature of a neonate is 101.5°F. It is equal to:

(A) 37.4°C.
(B) 37.7°C.
(C) 38.6°C.
(D) 39.0°C.

79c. A room temperature of 78°F is the same as:

(A) 23.3°C.
(B) 23.7°C.
(C) 24.4°C.
(D) 25.6°C.

Chapter

80

Tidal Volume Based on Flow and *I* Time

NOTES

The tidal volume delivered by a constant flow time-cycled ventilator is directly related to the flow rate and inspiratory time (*I* time), providing the peak inspiratory pressure is sufficient. A higher flow rate or longer *I* time usually yields a larger tidal volume in the absence of severe airway obstruction or lung parenchymal disease.

However, a prolonged *I* time increases the mean airway pressure and the likelihood of barotrauma. Therefore, as more ventilation is needed when using a constant flow time-cycled ventilator, one should evaluate and consider other options such as increasing the peak inspiratory pressure, ventilator frequency, or flow rate. Although these options carry similar complications, a combination of these options may help to improve ventilation with minimal side effects.

EQUATION

$V_T = \text{Flow} \times I \text{ time}$
V_T : Tidal volume in mL
Flow : Flow rate in mL/sec
I time : Inspiratory time in sec

EXAMPLE

Given: Flow $= 8$ L/min
       Inspiratory time $= 0.5$ sec
Calculate the approximate tidal volume.
First change the flow rate from L/min to mL/sec. Flow rate at 8 L/min is the same as 8,000 mL/60 sec or 133 mL/sec.

$$V_T = \text{Flow} \times I \text{ time}$$
$$= 133 \text{ mL/sec} \times 0.5 \text{ sec}$$
$$= 66.5 \text{ mL}$$

EXERCISE

Given the following settings on a pressure-limited ventilator: Flow = 6 L/min inspiratory time = 0.4 sec. What is the approximate tidal volume based on these settings?

[Answer: $V_T = 40$ mL]

REFERENCE

Whitaker

SEE

Mean Airway Pressure (MAWP).

SELF-ASSESSMENT QUESTIONS

80a. Given: flow = 7 L/min. inspiratory time = 0.5 sec. Calculate the delivered tidal volume based on these settings on a constant flow time-cycled ventilator.

(A) 45 mL
(B) 47 mL
(C) 50 mL
(D) 58 mL

80b. The following settings are used on a constant flow time-cycled ventilator: flow = 8 L/min, inspiratory time = 0.4 sec. Calculate the delivered tidal volume on these settings.

(A) 45 mL

(B) 47 mL

(C) 50 mL

(D) 53 mL

80c. Given the following flow rate (Flow) and inspiratory time (*I* time). Which set of values provides the lowest delivered tidal volume?

	Flow (L/min)	*I* time (sec)
(A)	7	0.3
(B)	7	0.4
(C)	6	0.4
(D)	6	0.5

80d. The following sets of data are found on the flow sheet of an infant ventilator over a 3-day period. Which set of values has the highest calculated tidal volume?

	Flow (L/min)	*I* time (sec)
(A)	7	0.5
(B)	8	0.4
(C)	6	0.5
(D)	7	0.4

80e. The physician asks a therapist to make changes on an infant ventilator so as to increase the tidal volume. The therapist should:

(A) decrease the F_IO_2.

(B) increase the inspiratory time.

(C) increase the *CPAP*.

(D) increase the expiratory time.

Chapter

81
Time Constant

NOTES

Time constant (*t*) is defined as the time needed to inflate a lung region to 60% of its filling capacity. It is directly related to the resistance (elastic lung parenchymal resistance and non-elastic airway resistance) and the compliance (lung and chest-wall compliance). When resistance and compliance are treated separately, an increase of time constant reflects an increase in resistance, or compliance, or both. Based on this equation, the lungs of a patient with high resistance or compliance take a longer time to inflate. Likewise, when the resistance and compliance are low, the time needed to inflate the lungs is shorter.

However, the relationship between resistance and compliance may mask the changes of time constant. For example, atelectasis causes a *decrease* in lung compliance but an *increase* in elastic lung parenchymal resistance. For this reason, opposing changes of compliance and resistance may result in an unchanged time constant.

A better way to evaluate the changes in resistance and compliance is to compare the dynamic and static compliance values.

During exhalation, an expiratory time equal to at least three time constants must be allowed if expiration is to reach 95%.

EQUATION

$t = R \times C$

t : Time constant in seconds
R : Resistance in cm H_2O/L/sec.
C : Compliance in L/cm H_2O

NORMAL VALUE

Use serial measurements to establish trend.

EXAMPLE

A patient who is on mechanical ventilation has a total resistance of 5 cm H_2O/L/sec and a compliance of 0.08 L/cm H_2O. What is the calculated time constant?

$t = R \times C$
$\quad = 5 \times 0.08$
$\quad = 0.4$ sec

EXERCISE

A patient who is being mechanically ventilated has a resistance of 6 cm H_2O/L/sec and a compliance of 0.06 L/cm H_2O. What is the calculated time constant?

[Answer: $t = 0.36$ sec.]

REFERENCES

Des Jardins; Wilkins (2)

SEE

Compliance: Dynamic (C_{dyn}); Compliance: Static (C_{st}).

SELF-ASSESSMENT QUESTIONS

81a. A patient who is on mechanical ventilation has a total resistance of 8 cm H_2O/L/sec and a compliance of 0.06 L/cm H_2O. What is the calculated time constant?

(A) 0.20 sec
(B) 0.48 sec
(C) 0.75 sec
(D) 1.33 sec

81b. A patient who is being mechanically ventilated has a total resistance of 7 cm H_2O/L/sec and a compliance of 0.033 L/cm H_2O. What is the calculated time constant?

(A) 0.15 sec
(B) 0.19 sec
(C) 0.23 sec
(D) 0.27 sec

81c. The pulmonary dynamics of a ventilator-dependent patient in the surgical intensive care unit are as follows: resistance = 12 cm H_2O/L/sec, compliance = 0.02 L/cm H_2O. What is the time constant based on the values provided?

(A) 0.06 sec
(B) 0.02 sec
(C) 0.2 sec
(D) 0.24 sec

Chapter

82

Vascular Resistance: Pulmonary

NOTES

Pulmonary vascular resistance (*PVR*) reflects the resistance of pulmonary vessel to blood flow. A Swan-Ganz catheter is required to obtain the $\overline{PA}$ and *PCWP* readings. The cardiac output must also be known to calculate the *PVR*.

The constant value 80 in the equation is used to convert the *PVR* to absolute resistance units, dynes · sec/cm^5.

Under normal conditions, the *PVR* is about one-sixth of the systemic vascular resistance. An abnormally high *PVR* may indicate pulmonary vascular problems, such as pulmonary hypertension, reduction of capillary bed, and pulmonary embolism. An extremely low *PVR* may be associated with reduction in circulating blood volume, such as hypovolemic shock.

See Tables 2-11 and 2-12 for factors that change the pulmonary vascular resistance.

EQUATION

$$PVR = (\overline{PA} - PCWP) \times \frac{80}{CO}$$

PVR	:	Pulmonary vascular resistance in dyne · sec/cm^5
$\overline{PA}$	:	Mean pulmonary artery pressure in mm Hg
PCWP	:	Pulmonary capillary wedge pressure in mm Hg
80	:	Conversion factor from mm Hg/L/min to dynes · sec/cm^5
CO	:	Cardiac output in L/min ($\dot{Q}_T$)

TABLE 2-11. Factors That Increase Pulmonary Vascular Resistance (*PVR*)

CHEMICAL STIMULI

Decreased alveolar oxygenation (alveolar hypoxia)

Decreased pH (acidemia)

Increased PCO_2 (hypercapnia)

PHARMACOLOGIC AGENTS

Epinephrine (Adrenalin®)

Norepinephrine (Levophed®, Levarterenol®)

Dobutamine (Dobutrex®)

Dopamine (Intropin®)

Phenylephrine (Neo-Synephrine®)

HYPERINFLATION OF LUNGS

Mechanical ventilation

Continuous Positive Airway Pressure (CPAP)

Positive End-Expiratory Pressure (*PEEP*)

PATHOLOGIC FACTORS

Vascular blockage

    Pulmonary emboli

    Air bubble

    Tumor mass

VASCULAR WALL DISEASE

Sclerosis

    Endateritis

    Polyarteritis

    Scleroderma

Vascular destruction

    Emphysema

    Pulmonary interstitial fibrosis

Vascular compression

    Pneumothorax

    Hemothorax

    Tumor mass

HUMORAL SUBSTANCES

Histamine

Angiotensin

Fibrinopeptides

Prostaglandin F$_{2\alpha}$

Serotonin

TABLE 2-12. Factors That Decrease Pulmonary Vascular Resistance (*PVR*)

PHARMACOLOGIC AGENTS	HUMORAL SUBSTANCES
Oxygen	Acetylcholine
Isoproterenol (Isuprel®)	Bradykinin
Aminophylline	Prostaglandin E
Calcium-blocking agent	Prostacyclin (prostaglandin I_2)

NORMAL VALUE $PVR = 50$ to 150 dyne $\cdot$ sec/cm^5

EXAMPLE   A patient has the following measurements. What is the calculated pulmonary vascular resistance (*PVR*)?

$\overline{PA}$ = 22 mm Hg
PCWP = 6 mm Hg
CO = 4.0 L/min

$$PVR = (\overline{PA} - PCWP) \times \frac{80}{CO}$$

$$= (22 - 6) \times \frac{80}{4.0}$$

$$= 16 \times \frac{80}{4.0}$$

$$= \frac{1280}{4}$$

$$= 320 \text{ dyne} \cdot \text{sec/cm}^5$$

EXERCISE   What is the patient's pulmonary vascular resistance (*PVR*) if the following measurements are recorded?

$\overline{PA}$ = 24 mm Hg
$PCWP$ = 7 mm Hg
CO = 5.0 L/min

[Answer: $PVR = 272$ dyne $\cdot$ sec/cm^5]

REFERENCE   Des Jardins

SEE   *Appendix Q: Hemodynamic Normal Ranges.*

SELF-ASSESSMENT QUESTIONS

82a. In order to calculate the pulmonary vascular resistance, all of the following measurements are required with the *exception* of:

(A) Systemic artery pressure.
(B) mean pulmonary artery pressure.
(C) pulmonary capillary wedge pressure.
(D) cardiac output.

82b. A patient has the following measurements: mean pulmonary artery pressure = 20 mm Hg, pulmonary capillary wedge pressure = 7 mm Hg, cardiac output = 5.0 L/min. What is the pulmonary vascular resistance (PVR)?

(A) 180 dynes · sec/cm^5

(B) 195 dynes · sec/cm^5

(C) 208 dynes · sec/cm^5

(D) 223 dynes · sec/cm^5

82c. The following hemodynamic measurements are obtained from a patient in the intensive care unit. What is the calculated pulmonary vascular resistance (PVR)?

Mean pulmonary artery pressure = 18 mm Hg

Pulmonary capillary wedge pressure = 8 mm Hg

Cardiac output = 4.5 L/min

(A) 146 dynes · sec/cm^5

(B) 155 dynes · sec/cm^5

(C) 160 dynes · sec/cm^5

(D) 178 dynes · sec/cm^5

82d. Calculate the patient's pulmonary vascular resistance (PVR) with the following measurements obtained during a hemodynamic study.

Mean pulmonary artery pressure = 20 mm Hg

Pulmonary capillary wedge pressure = 6 mm Hg

Cardiac output = 5.1 L/min

(A) 210 dynes · sec/cm^5

(B) 220 dynes · sec/cm^5

(C) 230 dynes · sec/cm^5

(D) 240 dynes · sec/cm^5

83

Vascular Resistance: Systemic

NOTES

Systemic vascular resistance (*SVR*) reflects the resistance of systemic vessel to blood flow. The *MAP* (mean arterial pressure) in the equation is a measured value, or it may be estimated by using the systolic and diastolic pressure readings (See *Mean Arterial Pressure*). The right atrial pressure and the cardiac output must also be known to calculate the *SVR*. The constant value 80 in the equation is used to convert the *SVR* to absolute resistance units dyne · sec/cm^5.

The normal *SVR* is about six times the pulmonary vascular resistance. An abnormally high *SVR* may indicate systemic vasoconstriction (e.g., response to hypovolemia). An abnormally low *SVR* may be indicative of peripheral vasodilation (e.g., early stages of septic shock).

See Table 2-13 for factors that change the systemic vascular resistance.

EQUATION

$$SVR = (MAP - \overline{RA}) \times \frac{80}{CO}$$

SVR : Systemic vascular resistance in dyne · sec/cm^5
MAP : Mean arterial pressure in mm Hg*
$\overline{RA}$: Mean right atrial pressure in mm Hg
80 : Conversion factor from mm Hg/L/min to dynes · sec/cm^5
CO : Cardiac output in L/min ($\dot{Q}_T$)

NORMAL VALUE

SVR = 800 to 1,500 dyne · sec/cm^5

EXAMPLE

A patient has the following measurements. What is the calculated systemic vascular resistance (*SVR*)?

MAP = 70 mm Hg
$\overline{RA}$ = 8 mm Hg
CO = 5.0 L/min

$$SVR = (MAP - \overline{RA}) \times \frac{80}{CO}$$

$$= (70 - 8) \times \frac{80}{5.0}$$

$$= 62 \times \frac{80}{5.0}$$

$$= \frac{4,960}{5}$$

$$= 992 \text{ dyne sec/cm}^5$$

EXERCISE

What is the patient's systemic vascular resistance (*SVR*) if the following measurements are recorded?

MAP = 76 mm Hg
$\overline{RA}$ = 6 mm Hg
CO = 5.0 L/min

[Answer: SVR = 1,120 dyne · sec/cm^5]

TABLE 2-13. Factors That Increase and Decrease Systemic Vascular Resistance (*SVR*)

INCREASES *SVR*	DECREASES *SVR*
Vasoconstricting Agents	**Vasodilating Agents**
Dopamine (Intropin®)	Nitroglycerin
Norepinephrine (Levarterenol®, Levophed®)	Nitroprusside (Nipride®)
	Morphine
Epinephrine (Adrenalin®)	Amrinone (Inocor®)
Phenylephrine (Neo-Synephrine®)	Hydralazine (Apresoline®)
	Methyldopa (Aldomet®)
Abnormal Conditions	Diazoxide (Hyperstat®)
Hypovolemia	
Septic shock (late stages)	**Abnormal Conditions**
↓ P_{CO_2}	Septic shock (early stages)
	↑ P_{CO_2}

↑ = *increased;* ↓ = *decreased.*

REFERENCE   Des Jardins

SEE   *See Mean Arterial Pressure; Appendix Q: Hemodynamic Normal Ranges.*

SELF-ASSESSMENT QUESTIONS

83a. To calculate a patient's systemic vascular resistance (*SVR*), all the following procedures or parameters are needed *except*:

   (A) pulmonary artery pressure.
   (B) mean arterial pressure.
   (C) mean right atrial pressure.
   (D) cardiac output.

83b. A patient has the following measurements: mean arterial pressure = 70 mm Hg, mean right atrial pressure = 10 mm Hg, cardiac output = 4.0 L/min. What is the systemic vascular resistance (*SVR*)?

   (A) 900 dynes · sec/cm^5
   (B) 1,000 dynes · sec/cm^5
   (C) 1,100 dynes · sec/cm^5
   (D) 1,200 dynes · sec/cm^5

83c. The following hemodynamic information is obtained from a patient's chart. What is the calculated systemic vascular resistance (*SVR*)?

   Mean arterial pressure = 62 mm Hg

   Mean right atrial pressure = 6 mm Hg

   Cardiac output = 4.2 L/min

   (A) 107 dynes · sec/cm^5
   (B) 667 dynes · sec/cm^5
   (C) 1,067 dynes · sec/cm^5
   (D) 1,120 dynes · sec/cm^5

83d. What is the patient's systemic vascular resistance (SVR) if the following measurements are recorded? $MAP = 55$ mm Hg, $\overline{RA} = 5$ mm Hg, $CO = 3.8$ L/min.

(A) 226 dynes · sec/cm^5

(B) 904 dynes · sec/cm^5

(C) 998 dynes · sec/cm^5

(D) 1,053 dynes · sec/cm^5

83e. The following hemodynamic measurements are obtained from a patient in the intensive care unit. What are the calculated pulmonary vascular resistance (PVR) and systemic vascular resistance (SVR)?

Mean pulmonary arterial pressure = 20 mm Hg

Pulmonary capillary wedge pressure = 7 mm Hg

Mean arterial pressure = 70 mm Hg

Mean right atrial pressure = 4 mm Hg

Cardiac output = 4.2 L/min

(A) $PVR = 226$ dynes · sec/cm^5; $SVR = 1{,}257$ dynes · sec/cm^5

(B) $PVR = 226$ dynes · sec/cm^5; $SVR = 1{,}303$ dynes · sec/cm^5

(C) $PVR = 248$ dynes · sec/cm^5; $SVR = 1{,}257$ dynes · sec/cm^5

(D) $PVR = 248$ dynes · sec/cm^5; $SVR = 1{,}303$ dynes · sec/cm^5

Chapter

84

Ventilator Rate Needed for a Desired $P_a CO_2$

Equation 1 assumes the following four conditions remain stable: metabolic rate (CO_2 production), ventilator tidal volume, spontaneous ventilation, and mechanical deadspace. The anatomic deadspace is not considered in this equation because it is an estimated value (by ideal body weight) and does not change significantly in practice.

If the ventilator tidal volume or mechanical deadspace is changed, use Equation 2.

If the ventilator tidal volume remains unchanged, new V_T = original V_T. If the mechanical deadspace remains unchanged, new V_D = original V_D.

EQUATION 1

$$\text{New rate} = \frac{\text{Rate} \times P_a CO_2}{\text{Desired } P_a CO_2}*$$

EQUATION 2

$$\text{New rate} = \frac{(\text{Rate} \times P_a CO_2) \times (V_T - V_D)}{\text{Desired } P_a CO_2 \times (\text{New } V_T - \text{New } V_D)}**$$

New rate	:	Ventilator rate needed for a desired $P_a CO_2$
Rate	:	Original ventilator rate/min
$P_a CO_2$	:	Original arterial carbon dioxide tension in mm Hg
Desired $P_a CO_2$	:	Desired arterial carbon dioxide tension in mm Hg
V_T	:	Original tidal volume
V_D	:	Original deadspace volume
New V_T	:	New tidal volume
New V_D	:	New deadspace volume

NORMAL VALUE

Set rate to provide eucapnic (patient's normal) ventilation.

EXAMPLE 1

When tidal volume and deadspace volume remain unchanged.

The $P_a CO_2$ of a patient is 55 mm Hg at a ventilator rate of 10/min. What should be the ventilator rate if a $P_a CO_2$ of 40 mm Hg is desired assuming the ventilator tidal volume and spontaneous ventilation are stable?

$$\begin{aligned}
\text{New rate} &= \frac{(\text{Rate} \times P_a CO_2)}{\text{Desired } P_a CO_2} \\
&= \frac{(10 \times 55)}{40} \\
&= \frac{550}{40} \\
&= 13.75 \text{ or } 14/\text{min}
\end{aligned}$$

*When tidal volume and deadspace volume stay unchanged.

**When tidal volume or deadspace volume is changed.

EXAMPLE 2

When tidal volume or deadspace volume is changed.

A patient has a P_aCO_2 of 25 mm Hg at a ventilator tidal volume of 800 mL, 0 mL added circuit deadspace, and a rate of 10/min. If the ventilator tidal volume is changed to 780 mL and if 50 mL of mechanical deadspace is added to the ventilator circuit, what should be the new ventilator rate for a desired P_aCO_2 of 40 mm Hg?

$$\text{New rate} = \frac{(\text{Rate} \times P_aCO_2) \times (V_T - V_D)}{\text{Desired } P_aCO_2 \times (\text{New } V_T - \text{New } V_D)}$$

$$= \frac{(10 \times 25) \times (800 - 0)}{40 \times (780 - 50)}$$

$$= \frac{(250) \times (800)}{40 \times (730)}$$

$$= \frac{200,000}{29,200}$$

$$= 6.85 \text{ or } 7/\text{min}$$

EXERCISE 1

At a ventilator rate of 8/min a patient's P_aCO_2 is 55 mm Hg. Calculate the new ventilator rate if a P_aCO_2 of 40 mm Hg is desired (assuming the ventilator tidal volume and spontaneous ventilation remain unchanged).

[Answer: New rate = 11/min]

EXERCISE 2

A patient has a P_aCO_2 of 30 mm Hg at a ventilator tidal volume of 700 mL and a rate of 8/min. If 50 mL of mechanical deadspace is added to the ventilator circuit, what should be the new ventilator rate for a desired P_aCO_2 of 40 mm Hg? What should be the calculated new rate if no mechanical deadspace is used?

[Answer: New rate = 6.46 or 7/min; new rate without deadspace = 6/min]

REFERENCES

Barnes; Burton

SELF-ASSESSMENT QUESTIONS

84a. Given: P_aCO_2 = 60 mm Hg, ventilator rate = 12/min. Calculate the estimated ventilator rate for a P_aCO_2 of 45 mm Hg (assuming the ventilator tidal volume and spontaneous ventilation are stable).

(12 × 60) × (

(A) 14/min
(B) 15/min
(C) 16/min
(D) 17/min

84b. Given: P_aCO_2 = 30 mm Hg, ventilator rate = 16/min. Calculate the estimated ventilator rate for a P_aCO_2 of 40 mm Hg (assuming the ventilator tidal volume and spontaneous ventilation are stable).

  (A) 11/min
  (B) 12/min
  (C) 13/min
  (D) 14/min

84c. The P_aCO_2 of a patient is 48 mm Hg at a ventilator rate of 12/min. What should be the ventilator rate if a P_aCO_2 of 36 mm Hg is desired (assuming the ventilator tidal volume and spontaneous ventilation are stable)?

  (A) 14/min
  (B) 15/min
  (C) 16/min
  (D) 17/min

84d. A patient has a P_aCO_2 of 22 mm Hg at a ventilator tidal volume of 850 mL and a rate of 12/min. If 50 mL of mechanical deadspace is added to the ventilator circuit, what should be the new ventilator rate for a desired P_aCO_2 of 35 mm Hg?

  (A) 7/min
  (B) 8/min
  (C) 9/min
  (D) 10/min

84e. A patient has a P_aCO_2 of 65 mm Hg at a ventilator tidal volume of 750 mL and a rate of 12/min. If the ventilator tidal volume is changed to 850 mL, what should be the new ventilator rate for a desired P_aCO_2 of 40 mm Hg?

  (A) 17/min
  (B) 16/min
  (C) 15/min
  (D) 14/min

84f. The P_aCO_2 of a patient is 28 mm Hg at a ventilator tidal volume of 900 mL and a rate of 16/min. If the ventilator tidal volume is decreased to 800 mL, what should be the new ventilator rate for a desired P_aCO_2 of 40 mm Hg?

  (A) 16/min
  (B) 15/min
  (C) 14/min
  (D) 13/min

Chapter

85

Weaning Index: Rapid Shallow Breathing (*RSBI*)

NOTES

Failure of weaning from mechanical ventilation may be related to a spontaneous breathing pattern that is rapid (high frequency) and shallow (low tidal volume). The ratio of spontaneous frequency and spontaneous tidal volume (in liters) has been used to evaluate the presence and severity of this breathing pattern.

Rapid shallow breathing is quantified as the f (breaths per minute) divided by the V_T in liters. This breathing pattern promotes inefficient, deadspace ventilation. When the f/V_T ratio becomes greater than 100 breaths/min/L, it suggests potential weaning failure. On the other hand, absence of rapid shallow breathing, as defined by an f/V_T ratio of less than 100 breaths/min/L, is a very accurate predictor of weaning success (Yang, 1991).

To measure the f/V_T ratio, the patient is taken off the ventilator and allowed to breathe spontaneously for at least one minute or until a stable breathing pattern has been established. Invalid assumption of the patient's breathing status may occur if measurements are done before the patient reaches a stable spontaneous breathing pattern. In addition, any ventilatory adjuncts such as mechanical ventilation (SIMV) or pressure support ventilation (PSV) should not be used in preparing the patient for the *RSBI* assessment.

EQUATION

$RSBI = f/V_T$

$RSBI$	:	Rapid Shallow Breathing Index, in breaths/min/L or cycles/L
f	:	Spontaneous frequency in breaths/min (cycles)
V_T	:	Spontaneous tidal volume, in liters

NORMAL VALUE

< 100 breaths/min/L is predictive of weaning success.

EXAMPLE

A patient who has been on mechanical ventilation is being evaluated for weaning trial. While breathing spontaneously, the minute ventilation is 4.5 L/min at a rate of 18/min. What is the average spontaneous tidal volume, in liters? What is the calculated Rapid Shallow Breathing Index (f/V_T)? Does this index suggest a successful weaning outcome?

Average spontaneous V_T = minute ventilation/frequency
$$= 4.5/18$$
$$= 0.25 \text{ L}$$

Rapid Shallow Breathing Index = f/V_T
$$= 18/0.25$$
$$= 72 \text{ breaths/min/L}$$

Because the Rapid Shallow Breathing Index is less than 100, the calculated index suggests a successful weaning outcome.

EXERCISE

A mechanically ventilated patient is being evaluated for weaning trial. The spontaneous minute ventilation and spontaneous frequency are 7.6 L/min and 36/min, respectively. What is the average spontaneous tidal volume, in liters? What is the calculated Rapid Shallow Breathing Index (f/V_T)? Does this index indicate a successful weaning outcome?

ANSWERS

Average spontaneous V_T = 0.21 L
Rapid Shallow Breathing Index = 171 breaths/min/L

As the Rapid Shallow Breathing Index is greater than 100 breaths/min/L, the calculated index suggests a poor weaning outcome.

The minute expired volume (V_E) is measured by a respirometer and the corresponding frequency (f) is recorded. The V_T is calculated by dividing the V_E by f. The f/V_T ratio is calculated by dividing the f by V_T. Remember, the V_T in the calculations is always expressed in liters.

REFERENCES   Tobin, 1986; Yang, 1991.

SELF-ASSESSMENT QUESTIONS

85a. Successful weaning from mechanical ventilation is likely when the *RSBI* is:

(A) greater than 100 breaths/min/L.
(B) less than 100 breaths/min/L.
(C) greater than 100 L.
(D) less than 100 L.

85b. *RSBI* requires measurements of the _____ minute ventilation and spontaneous _____.

(A) mechanical; frequency
(B) mechanical; tidal volume
(C) spontaneous; frequency
(D) spontaneous; tidal volume

85c. *RSBI* is calculated by:

(A) dividing a patient's spontaneous tidal volume by frequency.
(B) multiplying a patient's spontaneous tidal volume and frequency.
(C) dividing a patient's spontaneous frequency by tidal volume.
(D) multiplying a patient's spontaneous minute ventilation and frequency.

85d. Given the following measurements: Spontaneous minute ventilation = 4.5 L/min, spontaneous frequency = 23/min. What is the average spontaneous tidal volume, in liters?

(A) 0.196 L
(B) 0.511 L
(C) 1.96 L
(D) 5.11 L

85e. Given the following measurements: Spontaneous minute ventilation = 4.5 L/min, spontaneous frequency = 23/min. What is the calculated *RSBI*? Does the *RSBI* indicate a successful outcome?

(A) 110 breaths/min/L; Yes
(B) 110 breaths/min/L; No
(C) 117 breaths/min/L; Yes
(D) 117 breaths/min/L; No

85f. Given the following measurements: Spontaneous minute ventilation = 4.2 L/min, spontaneous frequency = 17/min. What is the average spontaneous tidal volume, in liters?

(A) 0.247 L

(B) 0.714 L

(C) 2.47 L

(D) 7.14 L

85g. Given the following measurements: Spontaneous minute ventilation = 4.2 L/min, spontaneous frequency = 17/min. What is the calculated *RSBI*? Does the *RSBI* indicate a successful outcome?

(A) 24 breaths/min/L; Yes

(B) 24 breaths/min/L; No

(C) 69 breaths/min/L; Yes

(D) 69 breaths/min/L; No

85h. Mr. Johns, a mechanically ventilated patient, is being evaluated for weaning attempt. His spontaneous minute ventilation and frequency are 5.9 L/min and 22/min, respectively. What is the average spontaneous tidal volume, in liters? What is the calculated Rapid Shallow Breathing Weaning Index (f/V_T)? Does the calculated *RSBI* suggest a successful weaning outcome?

(A) Average spontaneous V_T = 0.251 L; *RSBI* = 87 breaths/min/L; Yes

(B) Average spontaneous V_T = 0.268 L; *RSBI* = 82 breaths/min/L; Yes

(C) Average spontaneous V_T = 0.251 L; *RSBI* = 125 breaths/min/L; No

(D) Average spontaneous V_T = 0.268 L. *RSBI* = 125 breaths/min/L; No

85i. The spontaneous minute ventilation and frequency of a mechanically ventilated patient are 6.2 L/min and 30/min respectively. Calculate the average spontaneous tidal volume, in liters, and the Rapid Shallow Breathing Index (f/V_T). Does the calculated *RSBI* indicate a successful weaning outcome?

(A) Average spontaneous V_T = 0.207 L; *RSBI* = 90 breaths/min/L; Yes

(B) Average spontaneous V_T = 0.207 L. *RSBI* = 145 breaths/min/L; No

(C) Average spontaneous V_T = 0.219 L. *RSBI* = 90 breaths/min/L; Yes

(D) Average spontaneous V_T = 0.219 L. *RSBI* = 137 breaths/min/L; No

3

Ventilator Waveform

The ventilator waveforms presented in this section are for illustration purposes. Actual changes in the waveforms are influenced by other factors such as dual-mode settings and other co-existing patient conditions affecting the airflow resistance and lung compliance.

Contents

(6) Flow-Time Waveforms - Pressure-Controlled

Figure 3-18 Normal
Figure 3-19 Increased Resistance
Figure 3-20 Decreased Compliance

(7) Volume-Pressure Waveforms - Constant Flow

Figure 3-21 Normal
Figure 3-22 Increased Resistance
Figure 3-23 Decreased Compliance
Figure 3-24 Initial Point of Inflection (Ipi)
Figure 3-25 Point of Upper Inflection (Ipu)

(8) Flow-Volume Waveform

Figure 3-26 Decreased Airflow Resistance

Volume-Time Waveforms
Constant Flow

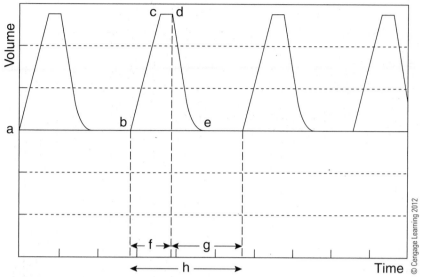

Figure 3-1 Normal
x-axis (time)
y-axis (volume)
a. baseline volume
b. beginning inspiration
c. end inspiration
b to c. inspiratory tidal volume
d. beginning expiration
c to d. inspiratory pause
e. end expiration
d to e. expiratory tidal volume
f. inspiratory time
g. expiratory time
h. respiratory cycle time

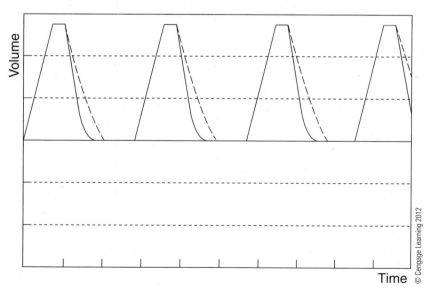

Figure 3-2 Increased Resistance
Solid line (normal)
Dotted line (increased resistance)
a. *slower* exponential decay to baseline volume (dotted line)
[*unchanged* inspiratory volume, pause time, expiratory volume, inspiratory time, expiratory time, and respiratory cycle time]

Volume-Time Waveforms
Constant Flow (contd)

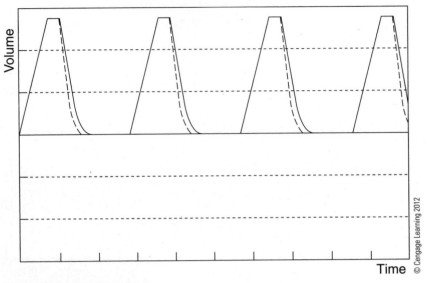

Figure 3-3 Decreased Compliance
Solid line (normal)
Dotted line (decreased compliance)
a. *faster* exponential decay to baseline volume (dotted line)
[unchanged inspiratory volume, pause time, expiratory volume, inspiratory time, expiratory time, and respiratory cycle time]

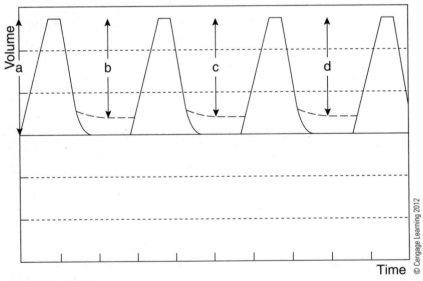

Figure 3-4 Air Leak
Solid line (normal)
Dotted line (air leak)
a. inspiratory tidal volume
b. expiratory tidal volume (expired volume < inspired volume)
c. expiratory tidal volume (expired volume < inspired volume)
d. expiratory tidal volume (expired volume < inspired volume)
[in air leaks, *every* expiratory tidal volume is less than the inspiratory tidal volume]

Volume-Time Waveforms
Constant Flow (contd)

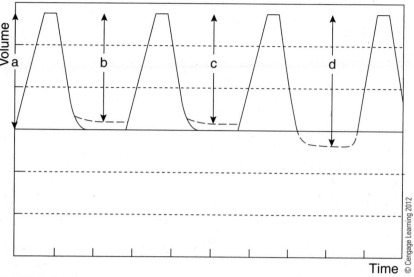

Figure 3-5 Air Trapping
Solid line (normal)
Dotted line (air trapping)
a. inspiratory tidal volume
b. expiratory tidal volume (expired volume < inspired volume)
c. expiratory tidal volume (expired volume < inspired volume)
d. expiratory tidal volume (expired volume > inspired volume)
[in air trapping, tidal volume *and* previously trapped air are exhaled every 2 to 3 breaths, resulting in an expired volume that is *larger* than the inspired volume]

Volume-Time Waveforms
Pressure-Controlled

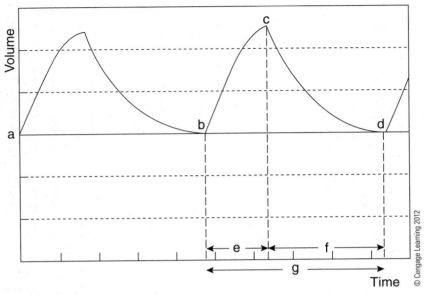

Figure 3-6 Normal
x-axis (time)
y-axis (volume)
a. baseline volume
b. beginning inspiration
c. end inspiration/beginning expiration
b to c. inspiratory tidal volume
d. end expiration
c to d. expiratory tidal volume
e. inspiratory time
f. expiratory time
g. respiratory cycle time

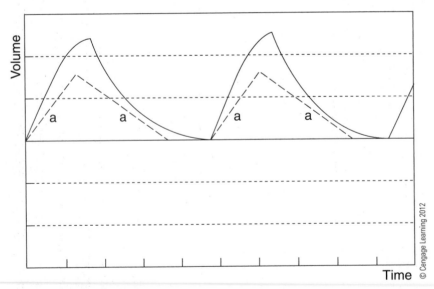

Figure 3-7 Increased Resistance
Solid line (normal)
Dotted line (increased resistance)
a. *smaller* inspiratory and expiratory tidal volumes (dotted line)

Volume-Time Waveforms
Pressure-Controlled (contd)

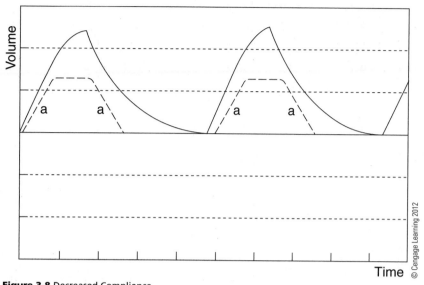

Figure 3-8 Decreased Compliance
Solid line (normal)
Dotted line (decreased compliance)
a. *smaller* inspiratory and expiratory tidal volumes (dotted line)

Pressure-Time Waveforms

Constant Flow

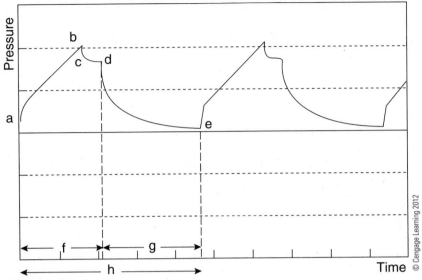

Figure 3-9 Normal
x-axis (time)
y-axis (pressure)
a. beginning inspiration
b. peak inspiratory pressure
c. beginning inspiratory pause
b to c. air flow resistance
d. end inspiratory pause/beginning expiration
c to d. plateau pressure (i.e., P_{PLAT}, static pressure)
e. end expiration
f. inspiratory time
g. expiratory time
h. respiratory cycle time

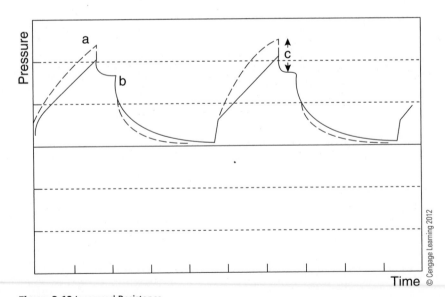

Figure 3-10 Increased Resistance
Solid line (normal)
Dotted line (increased resistance)
a. *higher* PIP
b. *unchanged* P_{PLAT}
c. larger difference between PIP and P_{PLAT}

Pressure-Time Waveforms
Constant Flow (contd)

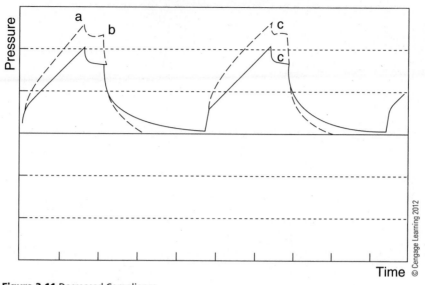

Figure 3-11 Decreased Compliance
Solid line (normal)
Dotted line (decreased compliance)
a. *higher* PIP
b. *higher* P_{PLAT}
c. unchanged difference between PIP and P_{PLAT} (a-b)

Pressure-Time Waveforms
Pressure-Controlled

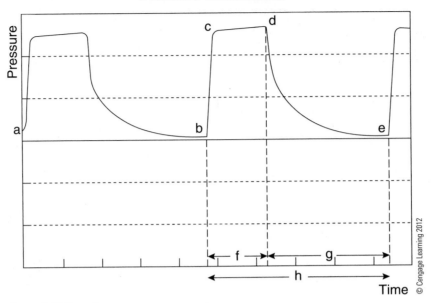

Figure 3-12 Normal
x-axis (time)
y-axis (pressure)
a. beginning inspiration
b. beginning inspiration/baseline pressure
c. peak inspiratory pressure
d. end inspiratory/beginning expiration
e. end expiration
f. inspiratory time
g. expiratory time
h. respiratory cycle time

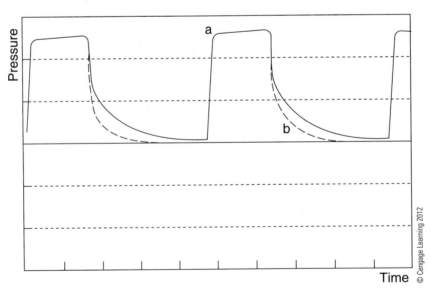

Figure 3-13 Increased Resistance
Solid line (normal)
Dotted line (increased resistance)
a. unchanged inspiratory phase
b. rapid decay to the second portion of pressure tracing

Pressure-Time Waveforms
Pressure-Controlled (contd)

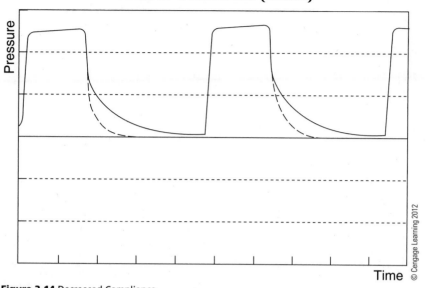

Figure 3-14 Decreased Compliance
Solid line (normal)
Dotted line (decreased compliance)
a. unchanged inspiratory phase
b. rapid decay of pressure tracing
c. expiratory pressure reaches baseline sooner

Flow-Time Waveforms
Constant Flow

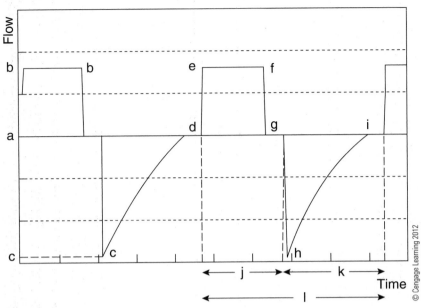

Figure 3-15 Normal
x-axis (time)
y-axis (flow)
a. baseline (separates inspiratory and expiratory flow patterns)
b. peak inspiratory flow
c. peak expiratory flow
d. beginning inspiration
e. peak inspiratory flow at beginning inspiration
f. peak inspiratory flow at end inspiration/beginning expiration
e to f. constant flow pattern
g. inspiratory pause
h. peak expiratory flow
i. end expiration (expiratory flow returns to baseline)
j. inspiratory time (includes pause time)
k. expiratory time (does *not* include pause time)
l. respiratory cycle time

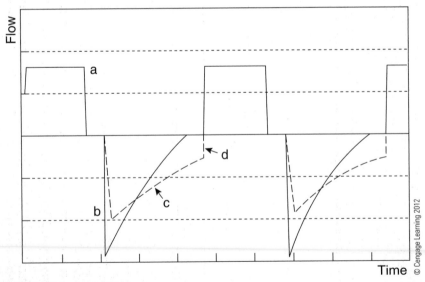

Figure 3-16 Increased Resistance
Solid line (normal)
Dotted line (increased resistance)
a. inspiratory phase does not change
b. *lower* expiratory flow as a result of increased airflow resistance during expiration
c. *slower* expiratory flow decay to baseline
d. air-trapping as expiratory flow does not reach baseline at end expiration (auto-*PEEP* may be observed in pressure-time waveform)

Flow-Time Waveforms
Constant Flow (contd)

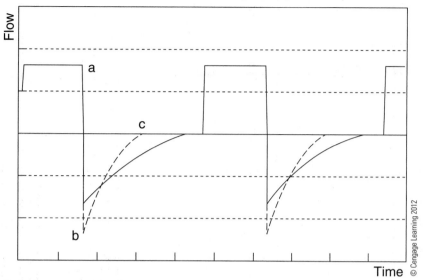

Figure 3-17 Decreased Compliance
Solid line (normal)
Dotted line (decreased compliance)
a. inspiratory phase does not change
b. *higher* peak expiratory flow as a result of increased lung recoil
(↑elastance/↓compliance)
c. *faster* expiratory flow decay to baseline as a result of increased lung recoil
(↑elastance/↓compliance)

Flow-Time Waveforms
Pressure-Controlled

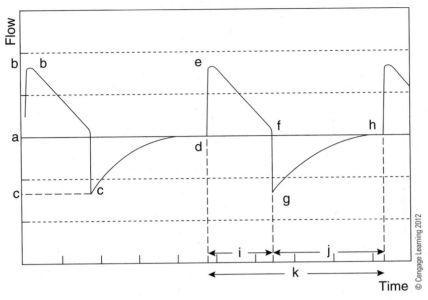

Figure 3-18 Normal
x-axis (time)
y-axis (flow)
a. baseline (separates inspiratory and expiratory flow patterns)
b. peak inspiratory flow
c. peak expiratory flow
d. beginning inspiration
e. peak inspiratory flow at beginning inspiration
f. inspiratory flow at end inspiration/beginning expiration
e to f. descending flow pattern
g. peak expiratory flow
h. end expiration (expiratory flow returns to baseline)
i. inspiratory time
j. expiratory time
k. respiratory cycle time

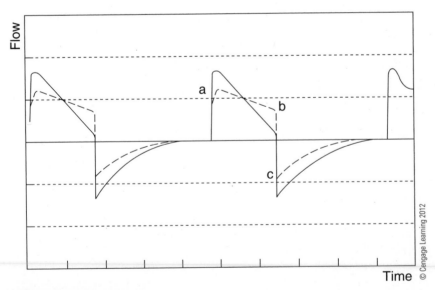

Figure 3-19 Increased Resistance
Solid line (normal)
Dotted line (increased resistance)
a. *lower* peak inspiratory flow
b. inspiratory flow stops before reaching baseline
c. *lower* peak expiratory flow

Flow-Time Waveforms
Pressure-Controlled (contd)

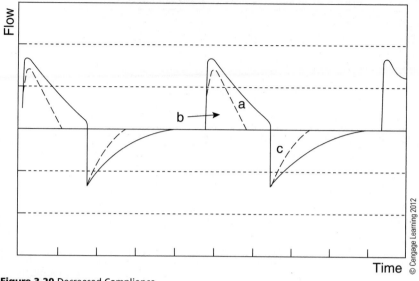

Figure 3-20 Decreased Compliance
Solid line (normal)
Dotted line (decreased compliance)
a. *faster* inspiratory flow decay to baseline before end of set inspiratory time
b. *lower* delivered tidal volume as a result of smaller flow-time area
c. *faster* expiratory flow decay to baseline as a result of increased lung recoil
(↑elastance/↓compliance)

Volume-Pressure Waveforms
Constant Flow

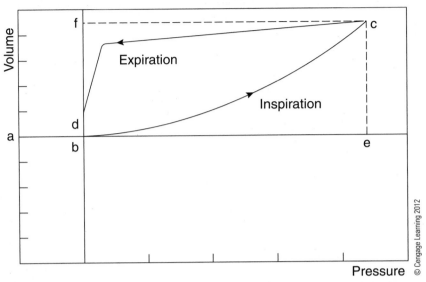

Figure 3-21 Normal
x-axis (pressure)
y-axis (volume)
a. baseline pressure/volume
b. beginning inspiration
c. end inspiration/beginning expiration
d. end expiration
e. peak inspiratory pressure
f. inspired volume (expired volume may differ in air leak or air trapping)

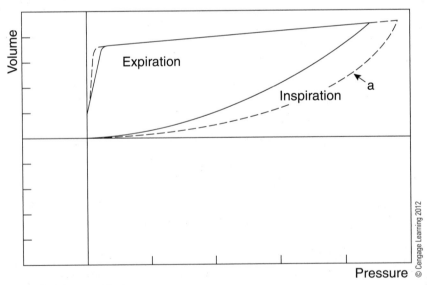

Figure 3-22 Increased Resistance
a. increase of pressure throughout the volume-pressure loop (inspiratory and expiratory phases)

Volume-Pressure Waveforms
Constant Flow (contd)

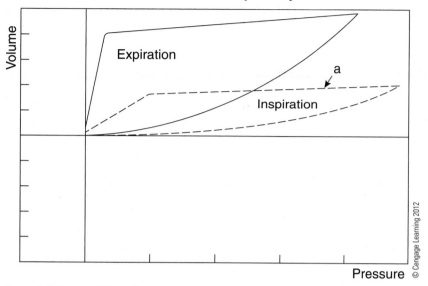

Figure 3-23 Decreased Compliance
a. shift of the volume-pressure loop toward the pressure-axis (usually x-axis)

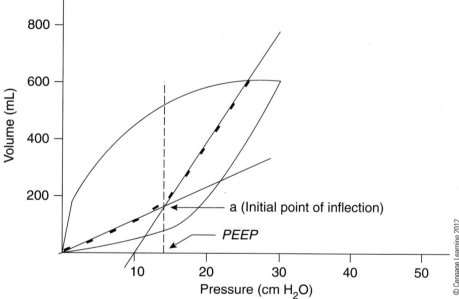

Figure 3-24 Initial Point of Inflection (Ipi)
a. change of slope from low compliance to improved compliance
[Because lung recruitment is likely to occur over the entire inspiratory inflation volume-pressure curve, the Ipi is only an approximation of the pressure at which the low compliance shows improvement. A *PEEP* level slightly higher than the Ipi (e.g., 2 cm H_2O) may be used initially to reduce the alveolar opening pressure.]

Volume-Pressure Waveforms
Constant Flow (contd)

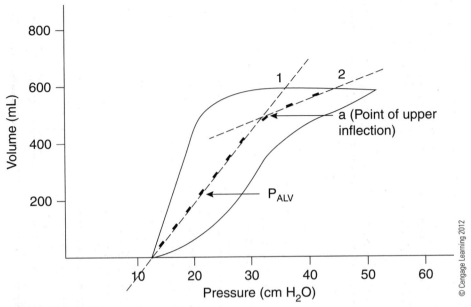

Figure 3-25 Point of Upper Inflection (Ipu)
a. change of slope from normal to reduced compliance as a result of overdistention of alveoli
[The Ipu is an approximation of the inspiratory pressure at which the compliance shows deterioration. The tidal volume may be reduced initially until the Ipu (duckbill) disappears, pending further evaluation of presence of overdistention.]

Flow-Volume Waveform

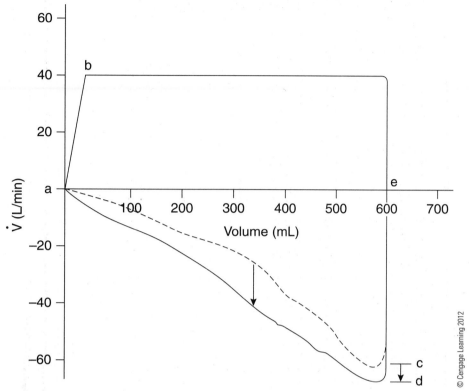

© Cengage Learning 2012

Figure 3-26 Decreased Airflow Resistance
x-axis (volume)
y-axis (+ inspiratory flow; − expiratory flow)
a. baseline flow/volume
b. peak inspiratory flow
c. abnormal peak expiratory flow (before bronchodilator)
d. normal peak expiratory flow (after bronchodilator)
c to d. improvement of peak expiratory flow (i.e., decreased airflow resistance)
e. tidal volume

4

Basic Statistics
and Educational Calculations

Statistics Terminology

Coefficient of Variation (CV)

Expresses the standard deviation as a percent of the mean:

$$CV = \left(\frac{s}{\overline{X}}\right) \times 100\%$$

The coefficient of variation (CV) is useful in comparing the dispersion of two or more sets of data measured by different instruments or methods. For example, if set A of measurements has a CV of 25% and set B of measurements has a CV of 14%, we can infer that the measuring instrument or method for set A has more random errors than that for set B. (See sample calculation in this section.)

Confidence Level

Probability level. The confidence level is usually set at 95% (0.05 level), which means that there is a 95% probability that the sample population is distributed in the same way as the whole population. For example, if statistical analysis provides a conclusion that is accepted at the 0.05 level, the researcher can be 95% confident that the conclusion can be applied to the whole population.

Control Group

A group of subjects whose selection and experiences are identical in every way possible to those of the treatment (experimental) group except that they do not receive the treatment.

Control Variable

A variable in the experimental design that is neutralized or canceled out by the researcher. This is the factor controlled by the researcher to neutralize any undesirable effect that might otherwise distort the observed outcome.

Correlation Coefficient (r)

Describes the relationship between two interval variables. It ranges from -1 (most negative relationship) to $+1$ (most positive relationship). For example, the coefficient may be positively related ($r = 0.86$) as in P_IO_2 and P_aO_2, or it may be negatively related ($r = -0.77$) as in alveolar ventilation and P_aCO_2.

If a regression line is constructed from the data points, it can "predict" one interval variable given the other interval variable.

Cut Score	The minimal passing score of an objective test or questionnaire. It is determined by a formula using the consensus of a group of subject-matter experts. (See sample calculation in this section.)
Dependent Variable	A response or output caused by the use of treatment or placebo. This is the factor observed and measured by the researcher to determine the effect of the independent variable.
Hypothesis	A suggested solution to a problem. It has the following characteristics: (1) It should have a statement based on logical derivation of a conclusion from facts; (2) it should be stated clearly and concisely in the form of a declarative sentence; and (3) it should be testable.
Independent Variable	A variable or input that operates within a person or an object that affects behavior or outcome. This is the factor selected and manipulated by the researcher to determine the relationship to an observed outcome.
Interval Variable	Lists the order of data and sets the distance between measurements. Heart rate, oxygen saturation, and drug dosages are interval variables because their measurements are equally spaced.
Kuder-Richardson Reliability Coefficient (K-R21)	A test reliability formula that is equivalent to the average of all possible split-half reliability coefficients. (See sample calculation in this section.)

$$K\text{-}R21 = 1 - \frac{\overline{X}(n - \overline{X})}{ns^2}$$

K-R21 = Kuder-Richardson reliability coefficient, Formula 21

$\overline{X}$ = Mean score on the test
n = Number of items in the test
s^2 = Test variance

Likert Scale	A five-point scale in which the intervals between successive measurements are equal. The Likert scale is often used in questionnaires because it can easily record the extent of agreement or disagreement with a statement.
Mean	The average measurement. It is computed by adding all measurements and then dividing by the number of measurements. (See sample calculation in this section.)
Median	The measurement in the middle of a ranked distribution; 50% of the measurements fall above it, and the other 50% fall below it. (See sample calculation in this section.)
Mode	The most frequently occurring measurement in a ranked distribution. If two measurements share the highest frequency count, the ranked distribution is called bimodal. (See example in this section.)

Nominal Variable	Also called categorical variable. The term "nominal" means "to name." A nominal variable classifies data into categories with no relation existing between the categories. For example, three categories of disease: chronic obstructive pulmonary disease, congestive heart failure, cystic fibrosis.
Null Hypothesis	A negative or "no differences" version of a hypothesis. When a null hypothesis is rejected, a significant difference between the two means is said to have occurred in a research study. (See *t*-test in this section.)
Ordinal Variable	The term "ordinal" means "to rank in order." An ordinal scale ranks data in terms of more than or less than. For example, no cyanosis, mild cyanosis, moderate cyanosis, severe cyanosis.
Placebo	An inert substance given to the control group in the same manner as to the treatment group. Placebos are often used in medical research to make it impossible for the subjects to determine whether they are receiving the active substance under study.
Range	The distance or measurement between the lowest and highest measurements. (See example in this section.)
Rating Scale	A device that can be used to summarize the observed activity. This scale may have three, five, seven, or an infinite number of points on a line with descriptive statements on both ends.
Ratio Scale	Data of physical science measurements including a true zero value such as blood pressure, arterial PO_2, height, and weight.
Reliability	Consistency. A *reliable* research study yields *consistent* results when the study is repeated. Reliability ranges from 0% (least reliable) to 100% (most reliable).
Revised Nedelsky Procedure	A three-step procedure to calculate the Cut Score of an evaluation instrument such as a multiple-choice exam. (See sample calculations in this section.)
Spearman-Brown Formula	A formula to calculate the whole test reliability (r_2). (See sample calculation in this section.) $$r_2 = \frac{n(r_1)}{1 + (n-1)r_1}$$ r_2 = whole test reliability n = number of parts (for halves, $n = 2$) r_1 = correlation coefficient
Split-Half Reliability	A reliability index of the internal consistency of a test that enables a researcher to determine whether the halves of a test are measuring the same quality or characteristic. The test is divided into halves, usually the odd-numbered items and the even-numbered items.

The correlation coefficient (r_1) is calculated by using the scores obtained by all students on one half of the exam and those obtained on the other half of the same exam. For a group of 30 students, 30 pairs of scores (30 scores for odd-numbered items and 30 scores for even-numbered items) would be used to calculate the correlation coefficient (r_1).

From the correlation coefficient (r_1), the whole test reliability (r_2) can be calculated by the Spearman-Brown formula.

Standard Deviation (s)

A measure of the spread or dispersion of a distribution of measurements. $N - 1$ in the equation is the degree of freedom. (See sample calculation in this section.) In text, the abbreviation for standard deviation is SD.

In the blood gas laboratory, standard deviation is used along with the mean to create a Levey-Jennings chart for graphic illustration of quality control results. Results falling within two standard deviations (± 2 SD) from the mean are considered "in control." Results falling outside two standard deviations from the mean are considered "out of control," and corrective actions must be taken to bring the results within two standard deviations.

Standard (z) Scores

A standard (z) score reflects the distance (in terms of standard deviations) of a measurement away from the mean. A z score of $+1.5$ means that the measurement is 1.5 standard deviations *above* the mean. A z score of -1.5 means that the measurement is 1.5 standard deviations *below* the mean. (See sample calculation in this section.)

t-test

The *t*-test allows a researcher to compare two means to determine the probability that the difference between the means is a real difference rather than a chance difference.

If the calculated t value is greater than the table t value at a specific confidence (p) level, then null hypothesis (i.e., that the means are equal) can be rejected at the p level. In other words, there is a statistical difference between the two means.

If the calculated t value is smaller than the table t value, there is no statistical difference between the means.

Treatment Group

A group of subjects whose selection and experiences are identical in every way possible to those of the control group. This is the group that receives the treatment.

Validity

The precision with which a research study measures what it purports to measure.

Variance (s^2)

The square of the standard deviation. (See example calculation in this section.)

REFERENCES

Chatburn; Gross; Nedelsky; Tuckman; White

Measures of Central Tendency

EXAMPLES 1-8	Ten scores from a 100-item final exam are ranked and listed as follows: 66, 66, 66, 73, 75, 79, 82, 84, 87, and 87. For examples 1 through 8, write or calculate the (1) range, (2) mode, (3) mean, (4) median, (5) standard deviation, (6) variance, (7) coefficient of variation, and (8) standard scores for 73 points and 82 points on the exam.
SOLUTION 1	*Range:* The range for the 10 exam scores is 66 to 87 points (21 points).
SOLUTION 2	*Mode:* The most frequently occurring measurement of these 10 exam scores is 66 points.
SOLUTION 3	*Mean $(\overline{X})$:*

$$\overline{X} = \frac{Sum\ of\ exam\ scores}{Number\ of\ scores}$$

$$= \frac{66 + 66 + 66 + 73 + 75 + 79 + 82 + 84 + 87 + 87}{10}$$

$$= \frac{765}{10}$$

$$= 76.5 \text{ points}$$

SOLUTION 4	*Median:* Because the median is the measurement in the middle of this ranked 10-number distribution, it falls between 75 (the fifth number) and 79 (the sixth number). The median is therefore

$$\frac{75 + 79}{2} = \frac{154}{2} = 77 \text{ points.}$$

SOLUTION 5

Standard Deviation (s):

Value of X	Mean ($\overline{X}$)	$(X - \overline{X})$	$(X - \overline{X})^2$
66	76.5	−10.5	110.25
66	76.5	−10.5	110.25
66	76.5	−10.5	110.25
73	76.5	−3.5	12.25
75	76.5	−1.5	2.25
79	76.5	2.5	6.25
82	76.5	5.5	30.25
84	76.5	7.5	56.25
87	76.5	10.5	110.25
87	76.5	10.5	110.25
		0	658.50

$$s = \sqrt{\frac{\text{Sum of } (X - \overline{X})^2}{\text{Degree of freedom}}}$$

$$= \sqrt{\frac{\text{Sum of } (X - \overline{X})^2}{(\text{Number of scores} - 1)}}$$

$$= \sqrt{\frac{\text{Sum of } (X - \overline{X})^2}{(N - 1)}}$$

$$= \sqrt{\frac{658.5}{(10 - 1)}}$$

$$= \sqrt{\frac{658.5}{9}}$$

$$= \sqrt{73.17}$$

$$= 8.554 \text{ points}$$

SOLUTION 6

Variance (s^2): Because variance is the square of the standard deviation, it is 73.17 (8.554^2).

SOLUTION 7

Coefficient of Variation (CV):

$$CV = \left(\frac{\text{standard deviation}}{\text{mean}} \right) \times 100\%$$

$$= \left(\frac{s}{\overline{X}} \right) \times 100\%$$

$$= \left(\frac{8.554}{76.5} \right) \times 100\%$$

$$= 0.1118 \times 100\%$$

$$= 11.18\%$$

SOLUTION 8

Standard (z) Scores: For a score of 73 points on the exam, the standard score (z) is calculated as follows:

$$z = \frac{X - \overline{X}}{s}$$

$$= \frac{73 - 76.5}{8.554}$$

$$= \frac{-3.5}{8.554}$$

$$= -0.41$$

The z score for 73 is 0.41 standard deviation *below* the mean. For a score of 82 points on the exam, the standard score (z) is calculated as follows:

$$z = \frac{X - \overline{X}}{s}$$

$$= \frac{82 - 76.5}{8.554}$$

$$= \frac{5.5}{8.554}$$

$$= 0.64$$

The z score for 82 is 0.64 standard deviation *above* the mean.

EXAMPLE 9

The mean and one standard deviation for a series of PO_2 calibration measurements are 157 mm Hg and ±3 mm Hg, respectively. If two standard deviations from the mean are used to set the limit of acceptance, which of the following six PO_2 calibration points is out of range? 155, 160, 153, 157, 164, 163 mm Hg.

SOLUTION 9

164 mm Hg is out of range.
A mean PO_2 of 157 mm Hg with one standard deviation (SD) of ±3 mm Hg would have two SD of ±6 mm Hg. Therefore, the acceptable range for PO_2 calibration is 151 (157 − 6) mm Hg to 163 (157 + 6) mm Hg. Of the six calibration points, 164 mm Hg is the only one outside this acceptable range.

EXAMPLE 10

The mean and one standard deviation for a series of normal pH calibration measurements are 7.375 and ±0.002, respectively. If measurements falling within two standard deviations from the mean are considered acceptable, which of the following seven pH calibration points is out of range? 7.379, 7.376, 7.374, 7.377, 7.370, 7375, and 7.376.

SOLUTION 10

7.370 is out of range.

A mean pH of 7.375 with one standard deviation (SD) of ±0.002 would have two SD of ±0.004. The acceptable range for pH calibration is therefore 7.371 (7.375 − 0.004) to 7.379 (7.375 + 0.004). Of the seven calibration points, 7.370 is the only one outside this acceptable range.

Exercises

EXERCISE 1-8

Nine mixed-venous oxygen content ($C_{\bar{v}}O_2$) measurements in volume percent (vol%) are ranked and listed as follows: 12, 14, 14, 15, 15, 16, 16, 16, and 17. Write or calculate the (1) range, (2) mode, (3) mean, (4) median, (5) standard deviation, (6) variance, (7) coefficient of variation, and (8) standard scores for 12 vol% and 16 vol%.

SOLUTION 1

Range: The range for the nine ($C_{\bar{v}}O_2$) measurements is 12 to 17 vol% (5 vol%).

SOLUTION 2

Mode: The most frequently occurring measurement of these nine $C_{\bar{v}}O_2$ values is 16 vol%.

SOLUTION 3

Mean ($\overline{X}$):

$$\overline{X} = \frac{\text{Sum of } C_{\bar{v}}O_2 \text{ measurements}}{\text{Number of measurements}}$$

$$= \frac{12 + 14 + 14 + 15 + 15 + 16 + 16 + 16 + 17}{9}$$

$$= \frac{135}{9}$$

$$= 15 \text{ vol}\%$$

SOLUTION 4

Median: Rank the nine numbers as follows: 12, 14, 14, 15, 15, 16, 16, 16, 17. As the median is the measurement in the middle of this ranked nine-number distribution, it falls between the fourth number and the sixth number. The median is therefore 15 vol%-the second 15 having four numbers before it and four numbers behind it.

SOLUTION 5   *Standard Deviation (s):*

Value of X	Mean $(\overline{X})$	$(X - \overline{X})$	$(X - \overline{X})^2$
12	1.5	−3	9
14	1.5	−1	1
14	1.5	−1	1
15	1.5	0	0
15	1.5	0	0
16	1.5	1	1
16	1.5	1	1
16	1.5	1	1
17	1.5	2	4
		0	18

$$s = \sqrt{\frac{\text{Sum of } (X - \overline{X})^2}{\text{Degree of freedom}}}$$

$$= \sqrt{\frac{\text{Sum of } (X - \overline{X})^2}{(\text{Number of } C_{\overline{v}}O_2 \text{ measurements} - 1)}}$$

$$= \sqrt{\frac{\text{Sum of } (X - \overline{X})^2}{(N - 1)}}$$

$$= \sqrt{\frac{18}{(9 - 1)}}$$

$$= \sqrt{\frac{18}{8}}$$

$$= \sqrt{2.25}$$

$$= 1.5 \text{ vol\%}$$

SOLUTION 6   *Variance (s^2):* As the variance is the square of the standard deviation, it is therefore 2.25 (1.5^2).

SOLUTION 7   *Coefficient of Variation (CV):*

$$CV = \left(\frac{\text{standard deviation}}{\text{mean}}\right) \times 100\%$$

$$= \left(\frac{s}{\overline{X}}\right) \times 100\%$$

$$= \left(\frac{1.5}{15}\right) \times 100\%$$

$$= 0.1 \times 100\%$$

$$= 10\%$$

SOLUTION 8   *Standard (z) Scores:* For 12 vol%, the standard score (z) is calculated as follows:

$$z = \frac{X - \overline{X}}{s}$$

$$= \frac{12 - 15}{1.5}$$

$$= \frac{-3}{1.5}$$

$$= -2$$

The *z* score for 12 vol% is 2 standard deviation *below* the mean.

For a score of 16, the standard score (*z*) is calculated as follows:

$$z = \frac{X - \overline{X}}{s}$$

$$= \frac{16 - 15}{1.5}$$

$$= \frac{1}{1.5}$$

$$= 0.67$$

The *z* score for 16 vol% is 0.67 standard deviation *above* the mean.

EXAMPLE 9

The mean and one standard deviation for a series of PO_2 calibration measurements are 102 mm Hg and ±1 mm Hg, respectively. If two standard deviations from the mean are used to set the limit of acceptance, which of the following five PO_2 calibration points is out of range? 102, 103, 99, 104, and 100 mm Hg.

SOLUTION 9

99 mm Hg is out of range.
A mean PO_2 of 102 mm Hg with one standard deviation (SD) of ±1 mm Hg would have two SD of ±2 mm Hg. Therefore, the acceptable range for PO_2 calibration is 100 (102 − 2) mm Hg to 104 (102 + 2) mm Hg. Of the five calibration points, 99 mm Hg is the only one outside this acceptable range.

EXAMPLE 10

The mean and one standard deviation for a series of acidotic pH calibration measurements are 7.135 and ±0.015, respectively. If measurements falling within two standard deviations from the mean are considered acceptable, which of the following six pH calibration points is out of range? 7.137, 7.165, 7.175, 7.125, 7,106, and 7.135.

SOLUTION 10

7.175 is out of range.
A mean pH of 7.135 with one standard deviation (SD) of ±0.015 would have two SD of ±0.030. The acceptable range for pH calibration is therefore 7.105 (7.135 − 0.030) to 7.165 (7.135 + 0.030). Of the six calibration points, 7.175 is the only one outside this acceptable range.

EXERCISE 11

The mean and one standard deviation for a series of PCO_2 calibration measurements are 44.9 mm Hg and ±0.5 mm Hg, respectively. Which of the following five PCO_2 calibration points (44.0, 45.6, 43.5, 45.0, and 46.5 mm Hg) is out of range if (A) *two* standard deviations from the mean are used to set the limit of acceptance; (B) *three* standard deviations from the mean are used to set the limit of acceptance.

SOLUTION 11

(A) 43.5 and 46.5 mm Hg are out of range; (B) 46.5 mm Hg is out of range.

(A) A mean PCO_2 of 44.9 mm Hg with one standard deviation (SD) of ± 0.5 mm Hg would have two SD of ± 1.0 mm Hg. Therefore, the acceptable range for PCO_2 calibration is 43.9 (44.9 − 1.0) mm Hg to 45.9 (44.9 + 1.0) mm Hg. Of the five calibration points, 43.5 mm Hg and 46.5 mm Hg are the PCO_2 measurements outside this acceptable range.

(B) If three standard deviations (± 1.5 mm 1 Hg) were used, the acceptable range for PCO_2 calibration would become 43.4 (44.9 − 1.5) mm Hg to 46.4 (44.9 + 1.5) mm Hg. Of the five calibration points, 46.5 mm Hg is the PCO_2 outside this acceptable range.

Test Reliability

Kuder-Richardson Reliability Coefficient (K-R21)

The Kuder-Richardson reliability coefficient calculates test reliability when the following are known: (1) mean score of the test, (2) variance of the test, and (3) number of items in the test. The reliability coefficient ranges from 0 (least reliable) to 1 (most reliable).

EXAMPLE

Ten scores from a 100-item final exam are ranked and listed as follows: 66, 66, 66, 73, 75, 79, 72, 84, 87, and 87. Calculate the reliability index of this exam using the Kuder-Richardson reliability coefficient (K-R21) formula. From previous examples, the mean (Example 3) and variance (Example 6) have been calculated and obtained. The reliability index may be calculated as follows:

$\overline{X}$ (mean score) $= 76.5$
n (number of items in the test) $= 100$
s^2 (variance) $= 73.17$

$$
\begin{aligned}
\text{K-R21} &= 1 - \frac{\overline{X}(n - \overline{X})}{ns^2} \\
&= 1 - \frac{76.5(100 - 76.5)}{100(73.17)} \\
&= 1 - \frac{76.5(23.5)}{7317} \\
&= 1 - \frac{1797.75}{7317} \\
&= 1 - 0.2457 \\
&= 0.7543 \text{ or } 75.43\%
\end{aligned}
$$

The test reliability based on the K-R21 formula is 75.43%.

EXERCISE 1

The mean score and variance of a 90-item exam are 72.8 and 66.2, respectively. Calculate the reliability of this exam using the Kuder-Richardson reliability coefficient (K-R21) formula.

SOLUTION 1

$\overline{X}$ (mean score)   = 72.8
n (number of items in the test) = 90
s^2 (variance)   = 66.2

$$K\text{-}R21 = 1 - \frac{\overline{X}(n - \overline{X})}{ns^2}$$

$$= 1 - \frac{72.8(90 - 72.8)}{90(66.2)}$$

$$= 1 - \frac{72.8(17.2)}{5958}$$

$$= 1 - \frac{1252.16}{5958}$$

$$= 1 - 0.2102$$

$$= 0.7898 \text{ or } 78.98\%$$

The test reliability based on the K-R21 formula is 78.98%.

EXERCISE 2

On a standardized 160-item comprehensive exam, the mean score and variance are 129.3 and 110.8, respectively. Use the Kuder-Richardson reliability coefficient (K-R21) formula to calculate the reliability of this exam.

SOLUTION 2

$\overline{X}$ (mean score)   = 129.3
n (number of items in the test) = 160
s^2 (variance)   = 110.8

$$K\text{-}R21 = 1 - \frac{\overline{X}(n - \overline{X})}{ns^2}$$

$$= 1 - \frac{129.3(160 - 129.3)}{160(110.8)}$$

$$= 1 - \frac{129.3(30.7)}{17728}$$

$$= 1 - \frac{3969.51}{17728}$$

$$= 1 - 0.2239$$

$$= 0.7761 \text{ or } 77.61\%$$

The test reliability based on the K-R21 formula is 77.61%.

SPEARMAN-BROWN FORMULA

The Spearman-Brown Formula calculates the whole test reliability when the correlation coefficient of the split-half scores is known. The split-half technique separates the exam into two halves, usually the odd-numbered and even-numbered exam items. Pairs of scores from the exam are then used to calculate the correlation coefficient. The whole test reliability index ranges from 0 (least reliable) to 1 (most reliable).

EXAMPLE

On a 60-item exam, the scores obtained by each student on the odd-numbered items and the even-numbered items are compared. The correlation coefficient (r_1) of the split-half technique is 0.67 for the entire class of 28 students (28 pairs of scores). Based on the information given, calculate the whole test reliability (r_2) with the Spearman-Brown formula.

r_2: whole test reliability
n (number of parts; for halves, $n = 2$) $= 2$
r_1 (correlation coefficient) $\qquad = 0.67$

$$r_2 = \frac{n(r_1)}{1 + (n - 1)r_1}$$

$$= \frac{2(0.67)}{1 + (2 - 1)0.67}$$

$$= \frac{1.34}{1 + (1)0.67}$$

$$= \frac{1.34}{1 + 0.67}$$

$$= \frac{1.34}{1.67}$$

$$= 0.8024 \text{ or } 80.24\%$$

The whole test reliability based on the Spearman-Brown formula is 80.24%.

EXERCISE 1

A 90-item exam was given to a class of 34 students. The 34 pairs of scores were obtained by splitting and scoring the exam by odd-numbered and even-numbered items. The correlation coefficient (r_1) for the 34 pairs of scores by this split-half technique is 0.58.

Based on the information given, calculate the whole test reliability (r_2) with the Spearman-Brown formula.

SOLUTION 1

r_2: whole test reliability
n (number of parts; for halves, $n = 2$) $= 2$
r_1 (correlation coefficient) $\qquad = 0.58$

$$r_2 = \frac{n(r_1)}{1 + (n - 1)r_1}$$

$$= \frac{2(0.58)}{1 + (2 - 1)0.58}$$

$$= \frac{1.16}{1 + (1)0.58}$$

$$= \frac{1.16}{1 + 0.58}$$

$$= \frac{1.16}{1.58}$$

$$= 0.7342 \text{ or } 73.42\%$$

The whole test reliability based on the Spearman-Brown formula is 73.42%.

EXERCISE 2

Twenty pairs of scores are recorded from a 60-item exam administered to a class of 20 students. Each pair of scores represents the number of correct answers obtained by each student from the odd-numbered and even-numbered exam items. The correlation coefficient (r_1) for the 20 pairs of scores is 0.75. Based on the information given, what is the calculated whole test reliability (r_2) with the Spearman-Brown formula?

SOLUTION 2

r_2: whole test reliability
n (number of parts; for halves, $n = 2$) = 2
r_1 (correlation coefficient) = 0.75

$$r_2 = \frac{n(r_1)}{1 + (n-1)r_1}$$

$$= \frac{2(0.75)}{1 + (2-1)0.75}$$

$$= \frac{1.5}{1 + (1)0.75}$$

$$= \frac{1.5}{1 + 0.75}$$

$$= \frac{1.5}{1.75}$$

$$= 0.8571 \text{ or } 85.71\%$$

The whole test reliability based on the Spearman-Brown formula is 85.71%.

Cut Score: Revised Nedelsky Procedure

In 1954, Leo Nedelsky published a procedure to compute the cut score (minimum passing score) of a multiple-choice exam. Among other factors that make an exam item "difficult" or "easy," the Nedelsky procedure accounts for the degree of difficulty of the distractors in a multiple-choice exam item.

The original procedure was revised by Leon J. Gross in 1985. In this revised procedure, a three-point distribution (0 to 2) is used. The revised procedure by Gross is summarized as follows.

STEP 1 — All responses to a multiple-choice exam item are evaluated by a group of subject-matter experts. Consensus is then obtained from these experts, and points ranging from 0 to 2 are assigned to each response.

The one *correct response* is scored *2 points* (weight of correct response).

Each *plausible but incorrect response* is scored *1 point* (weight of plausible, incorrect response). This represents an "acceptable" error for the minimally competent examinee.

Each *implausible and incorrect response* is scored *0 points* (weight of implausible, incorrect response). This represents an unacceptable error that should have been avoided even by the minimally competent examinee.

STEP 2 — The minimal pass index (MPI) for each exam item is calculated by:

$$MPI = \frac{\text{Weight of correct response}}{\text{Sum of all weights for each item}}$$

STEP 3 — Cut score = MPI of all exam items $\times$ 95%.

A value of 95% is used to avoid extreme cut scores in the original Nedelsky procedure. This value may be adjusted up or down depending on the degree of chance and perfection (number of responses) in each exam item.

EXAMPLE 1 — Find the minimal pass index (MPI) of the multiple-choice exam item below.

Under normal tidal volume and respiratory rate, the P_1O_2 provided by a nasal cannula at 2 L/min of oxygen is about

A. 21%
B. 24%
C. 28%
D. 32%

STEP 1

The four responses are evaluated by a group of experts. Their consensus and point assignments to each response are as follows.

A. 21%:   0 points
B. 24%:   1 point
C. 28%:   2 points
D. 32%:   1 point

Response (A) is scored 0 points because even the minimally competent examinee should be able to eliminate this option since the P_1O_2 provided by a nasal cannula at 2 L/min of oxygen must be greater than 21% (P_1O_2 of room air).

Responses (B) and (D) are scored 1 point each because they are incorrect but plausible responses.

Response (C) is scored 2 points because it is the correct response.

STEP 2

The minimal pass index (MPI) of this exam item is therefore:

$$MPI = \frac{\text{Weight of correct response}}{\text{Sum of all weights for item}}$$

$$= \frac{2 \text{ points}}{(0 + 1 + 2 + 1) \text{ points}}$$

$$= \frac{2}{4}$$

$$= 0.5$$

EXAMPLE 2

Calculate the cut score of a 10-item multiple-choice exam with the following minimal pass indices (MPI) for the 10 exam items: 0.67, 0.5, 1.0, 0.67, 0.4, 0.5, 0.4, 0.67, 0.5, and 1.0.

$$\text{Cut score} = \text{MPI of all exam items} \times 95\%$$

$$= (0.67 + 0.5 + 1.0 + 0.67 + 0.4 + 0.5$$

$$+ 0.4 + 0.67 + 0.5 + 1.0) \times 95\%$$

$$= 6.31 \times 95\%$$

$$= 5.99 \text{ or } 6 \text{ points}$$

The cut score (minimal passing score) of this 10-item multiple-choice exam is 6 points.

EXERCISE 1

As shown below, the point assignments for each response to an exam item are provided by a group of experts. What is the minimal pass index (MPI) of this exam item?

The preferred puncture site for arterial blood gas sampling in an adult is the:

A. radial artery: 2 points
B. umbilical artery: 0 points
C. brachial artery: 1 point
D. coronary artery: 0 points

SOLUTION 1

$$\text{MPI} = \frac{\text{Weight of correct response}}{\text{Sum of all weights for item}}$$

$$= \frac{2 \text{ points}}{3 \text{ points}}$$

$$= 0.67$$

EXERCISE 2

Use the revised Nedelsky procedure to calculate the cut score of a nine-item multiple-choice exam with the following minimal pass indices for the nine exam items: 0.5, 1.0, 0.67, 0.4, 0.4, 0.67, 0.5, 0.67, and 0.4.

SOLUTION 2

$$\begin{aligned} \text{Cut score} &= \text{MPI of all exam items} \times 95\% \\ &= (0.5 + 1.0 + 0.67 + 0.4 + 0.4 + 0.67 + 0.5 \\ &\quad + 0.67 + 0.4) \times 95\% \\ &= 5.21 \times 95\% \\ &= 4.95 \text{ or } 5 \text{ points} \end{aligned}$$

EXERCISE 3

If the sum of all minimal pass indices (MPI) in a 98-item multiple-choice exam is 81, what is the cut score using the revised Nedelsky procedure?

SOLUTION 3

$$\begin{aligned} \text{Cut score} &= \text{MPI of all exam items} \times 95\% \\ &= 81 \times 95\% \\ &= 76.95 \text{ or } 77 \text{ points} \end{aligned}$$

REFERENCES

Gross; Nedelsky

5

Answer Key
to Self-Assessment Questions

Question no.	Answer	Question no.	Answer
1a	(A)	12a	(B)
1b	(B)	12b	(A)
1c	(B)	12c	(B)
		12d	(C)
2a	(D)	12e	(D)
2b	(D)		
2c	(C)	13a	(C)
2d	(B)	13b	(B)
		13c	(C)
3a	(A)	13d	(C)
3b	(D)		
3c	(C)	14a	(A)
3d	(D)	14b	(D)
		14c	(B)
4a	(C)	14d	(B)
4b	(D)	14e	(C)
4c	(B)		
4d	(D)	15a	(A)
4e	(A)	15b	(B)
		15c	(D)
5a	(A)	15d	(D)
5b	(B)		
5c	(C)	16a	(D)
5d	(C)	16b	(D)
		16c	(B)
6a	(D)		
6b	(A)	17a	(D)
6c	(D)	17b	(C)
		17c	(D)
7a	(A)	17d	(C)
7b	(D)	17e	(D)
7c	(C)	17f	(B)
7d	(C)	17g	(A)
8a	(C)	18a	(A)
8b	(B)	18b	(D)
8c	(D)	18c	(D)
8d	(A)	18d	(C)
9a	(C)	19a	(C)
9b	(A)	19b	(A)
9c	(A)	19c	(D)
		19d	(D)
10a	(C)	19e	(C)
10b	(B)	19f	(D)
10c	(A)	19g	(A)
10d	(A)		
10e	(C)	20a	(C)
10f	(A)	20b	(A)
		20c	(D)
11a	(D)	20d	(A)
11b	(D)	20e	(D)
11c	(A)		
11d	(C)	21a	(B)
		21b	(D)

Question no.	Answer	Question no.	Answer
21c	(A)	29c	(D)
21d	(B)	29d	(B)
22a	(D)	30a	(D)
22b	(C)	30b	(D)
22c	(D)	30c	(A)
22d	(B)	30d	(B)
22e	(C)	30e	(D)
23a	(C)	31a	(D)
23b	(A)	31b	(C)
23c	(C)	31c	(B)
23d	(D)	31d	(D)
23e	(A)	31e	(B)
23f	(C)		
23g	(D)	32a	(C)
23h	(C)	32b	(A)
23i	(D)	32c	(A)
24a	(C)	33a	(D)
24b	(C)	33b	(C)
24c	(B)	33c	(B)
24d	(C)		
24e	(D)	34a	(D)
24f	(D)	34b	(A)
24g	(A)	34c	(B)
24h	(B)		
24i	(C)	35a	$FEV_1 = 0.75$ L,
24j	(A)		$FVC = 3.5$ L,
24k	(D)		$FEV_1\% = 21.4\%$,
24l	(A)		$FEV_1\%$ is abnormal
24m	(B)	35b	$FEV_2 = 2.15$ L,
			$FVC = 4.5$ L,
25a	(B)		$FEV_2\% = 47.8\%$,
25b	(C)		$FEV_2\%$ is abnormal
25c	(C)	35c	$FEV_3 = 4.0$ L,
25d	(A)		$FVC = 5.5$ L,
			$FEV_3\% = 72.7\%$,
26a	(A)		$FEV_3\%$ is abnormal
26b	(C)		
26c	(C)	36a	$FEF_{200-1200} = 0.6$ L/sec
		36b	$FEF_{200-1200} = 1.1$ L/sec
27a	(D)	36c	$FEF_{200-1200} = 1.8$ L/sec
27b	(C)		
27c	(A)	37a	$FEF_{25-75}\% = 0.5$ L/sec
27d	(D)	37b	$FEF_{25-75}\% = 0.75$ L/sec
		37c	$FEF_{25-75}\% = 1.15$ L/sec
28a	(A)		
28b	(C)	38a	(D)
28c	(B)	38b	(C)
28d	(D)	38c	(A)
		38d	(C)
29a	(B)	38e	(C)
29b	(C)	38f	(B)

Question no.	Answer		Question no.	Answer
38g	(C)		45e	(D)
38h	(B)		45f	(A)
38i	(C)		45g	(B)
38j	(C)		45h	(B)
			45i	(D)
39a	(D)		45j	(C)
39b	(A)		45k	(A)
39c	(D)		45l	(C)
39d	(D)		45m	(D)
			45n	(D)
40a	(C)		45o	(D)
40b	(A)		45p	(C)
40c	(D)		45q	(A)
			45r	(C)
41a	(D)		45s	(B)
41b	(C)		45t	(B)
41c	(D)			
41d	(B)		46a	(A)
			46b	(C)
42a	(B)		46c	(D)
42b	(A)		46d	(B)
42c	(C)		46e	(C)
			46f	(B)
43a	(C)			
43b	(C)		47a	(A)
43c	(A)		47b	(C)
43d	(D)		47c	(B)
43e	(A)		47d	(D)
43f	(A)		47e	(B)
43g	(D)		47f	(C)
43h	(D)		47g	(C)
43i	(C)			
43j	(A)		48a	(B)
43k	(B)		48b	(D)
43l	(C)		48c	(C)
43m	(B)		48d	(D)
43n	(D)			
43o	(A)		49a	(B)
43p	(A)		49b	(D)
43q	(D)		49c	(C)
43r	(A)		49d	(A)
43s	(D)		49e	(C)
43t	(D)		49f	(D)
43u	(B)		49g	(B)
			49h	(C)
44a	(A)			
44b	(B)		50a	(C)
44c	(B)		50b	(B)
44d	(C)		50c	(C)
			50d	(C)
45a	(C)		50e	(D)
45b	(D)		50f	(A)
45c	(A)		50g	(B)
45d	(A)		50h	(D)

Question no.	Answer	Question no.	Answer
51a	(C)	56k	(B)
51b	(C)	56l	(D)
51c	(A)		
51d	(D)	57a	(C)
51e	(B)	57b	(B)
51f	(B)	57c	(C)
51g	(D)	57d	(A)
51h	(C)	57e	(D)
51i	(A)		
		58a	(A)
52a	(D)	58b	(D)
52b	(C)	58c	(A)
52c	(B)	58d	(A)
53a	(B)	59a	(D)
53b	(C)	59b	(C)
53c	(D)	59c	(C)
53d	(C)	59d	(A)
53e	(C)	59e	(A)
53f	(D)		
53g	(C)	60a	(C)
53h	(B)	60b	(C)
53i	(B)	60c	(D)
53j	(D)	60d	(B)
53k	(C)	60e	(D)
53l	(B)	60f	(A)
53m	(B)	60g	(A)
54a	(B)	61a	(B)
54b	(A)	61b	(D)
54c	(B)	61c	(D)
54d	(C)	61d	(D)
54e	(D)	61e	(C)
54f	(C)	61f	(B)
54g	(D)	61g	(A)
		61h	(C)
55a	(A)	61i	(A)
55b	(C)	61j	(C)
55c	(D)	61k	(C)
55d	(D)		
55e	(B)	62a	(C)
55f	(A)	62b	(D)
55g	(B)	62c	(A)
		62d	(D)
56a	(C)		
56b	(C)	63a	(D)
56c	(D)	63b	(B)
56d	(A)	63c	(C)
56e	(A)	63d	(A)
56f	(B)		
56g	(B)	64a	(B)
56h	(C)	64b	(A)
56i	(C)	64c	(D)
56j	(D)	64d	(C)

Question no.	Answer	Question no.	
65a	(C)	73a	
65b	(A)	73b	
65c	(D)	73c	
65d	(C)		
65e	(D)	74a	
65f	(B)	74b	(D)
65g	(A)	74c	(D)
65h	(B)	74d	(D)
65i	(D)	74e	(B)
66a	(D)	75a	(B)
66b	(C)	75b	(C)
66c	(C)	75c	(C)
66d	(C)	75d	(A)
		75e	(C)
67a	(C)		
67b	(D)	76a	(C)
67c	(B)	76b	(D)
		76c	(B)
68a	(B)	76d	(A)
68b	(A)	76e	(D)
68c	(B)	76f	(B)
68d	(C)		
68e	(D)	77a	(C)
		77b	(D)
69a	(C)	77c	(A)
69b	(B)	77d	(C)
69c	(D)		
		78a	(B)
70a	(A)	78b	(C)
70b	(D)	78c	(D)
70c	(D)	78d	(C)
70d	(C)	78e	(B)
71a	(A)	79a	(B)
71b	(D)	79b	(C)
71c	(B)	79c	(D)
71d	(B)		
71e	(A)	80a	(D)
71f	(C)	80b	(D)
71g	(D)	80c	(A)
71h	(B)	80d	(A)
71i	(C)	80e	(B)
71j	(C)		
71k	(A)	81a	(B)
		81b	(C)
72a	(C)	81c	(D)
72b	(C)		
72c	(B)	82a	(A)
72d	(D)	82b	(C)
72e	(B)	82c	(D)
72f	(C)	82d	(B)
72g	(C)		
72h	(A)	83a	(A)
72i	(A)	83b	(D)

Question no.	Answer	Question no.	Answer
83c	(C)	85a	(B)
83d	(D)	85b	(C)
83e	(C)	85c	(C)
		85d	(A)
84a	(C)	85e	(D)
84b	(B)	85f	(A)
84c	(C)	85g	(C)
84d	(B)	85h	(B)
84e	(A)	85i	(B)
84f	(D)		

6

Symbols and Abbreviations

Symbols and Abbreviations Commonly Used in Respiratory Physiology

Primary Symbols

GAS SYMBOLS

P Pressure

V Gas volume

$\dot{V}$ Gas volume per unit of time, or flow

F Fractional concentration of gas

BLOOD SYMBOLS

O Blood volume

$\dot{Q}$ Blood flow

C Content in blood

S Saturation

Secondary Symbols

GAS SYMBOLS

I   Inspired

E   Expired

A   Alveolar

T   Tidal

D   Deadspace

BLOOD SYMBOLS

a   Arterial

c   Capillary

v   Venous

$\bar{v}$ Mixed venous

Abbreviations

%:   Percent

$\%_g$:   Percent of gas in the mixture

a/A ratio: Arterial/alveolar oxygen tension ratio in %

BD: Base deficit in mEq/L, negative base excess (–BE)

$BP_{systolic}$:   Systolic blood pressure in mm Hg

$BP_{diastolic}$:   Diastolic blood pressure in mm Hg

BSA: Body surface area in m^2

C: Compliance in mL/cm H_2O or L/cm H_2O

°C: degree Celsius

C_{dyn}:   Dynamic compliance in mL/cm H_2O

C_{st}:   Static compliance in mL/cm H_2O

C_aO_2:   Arterial oxygen content in vol%

Capacity: Maximum amount of water that air can hold at a given temperature in mg/L or mm Hg

$C_{(a-\bar{v})}O_2$:   Arterial-mixed venous oxygen content difference in vol%

C_cO_2:   End-capillary oxygen content in vol%

CI: Cardiac index in L/min/m^2

Cl^-:   Serum chloride concentration in mEq/L

cm H_2O: Centimeters of water, a unit of pressure measurement

CO: Cardiac output in L/min ($\dot{Q}_T$)

$C_{\bar{v}}O_2$:   Mixed venous oxygen content in vol%

D: Density of gas in g/L

dyne · sec/cm^5:   dyne · second/centimeter^5, a vascular resistance unit

E: Elastance in cm H_2O/L

ERV: Expiratory reserve volume in mL or L

Expired V_T: Expired tidal volume in mL or L

°F: degree Fahrenheit

f: Frequency per minute; respiratory rate

f_{MECH}:   Mechanical ventilator frequency rate per minute

f_{SPON}:   Patient's spontaneous frequency rate per minute

°FEF_{25-75}%:   Forced Expiratory Flow of the middle 50% of vital capacity

$FEF_{200-1,200}$:   Forced Expiratory Flow of 200 to 1,200 mL of vital capacity

FEV_t: Forced Expiratory Volume (timed)

FEV_t%:   Forced Expiratory Volume (timed percent)

F_IO_2:   Inspired oxygen concentration in %

Flow: Flow rate in L/sec or L/min

FRC: Functional residual capacity in mL or L

g: gram

g · m/beat: gram · meter/beat, a ventricular stroke work unit

g · m/beat/m^2:   gram · meter/beat/meter^2, a ventricular stroke work index unit

gmw: Gram molecular weight in g

HCO_3^-:   (1) Serum bicarbonate concentration in mEq/L
      (2) Sodium bicarbonate needed to correct base deficit, in mEq/L

H_2CO_3:   Carbonate acid in mEq/L

Hb: Hemoglobin content in g%

HD: Humidity deficit in mg/L

HR: Heart rate per minute

IC: Inspiratory capacity in mL or L

ID: Internal diameter of endotracheal tube in mm

I time: Inspiratory time in sec

IRV: Inspiratory reserve volume in mL or L

°K: Kelvin

kg: Body weight in kilograms

kPa: International System (SI) unit for pressure (kilopascal); 1 kPa equals 7.5 torr
      or mm Hg

L: Liter

L/min: Liters per minute; LPM

log: logarithm

LPM: Liters per minute; L/min

LVSW: Left ventricular stroke work in g · m/beat

LVSWI: Left ventricular stroke work index in g · m/beat/m^2

MAP: Mean arterial pressure in mm Hg

MAWP: Mean airway pressure in cm H_2O ($\overline{P}_{aw}$)

min: Minute

mL: Milliliter

mm Hg: Millimeters of mercury, a unit of pressure measurement (torr);
      equal to 0.1333 kPa

Na^+:   Serum sodium concentration in mEq/L

O_2:air: Oxygen:air entrainment ratio

O_2 consumption: Estimated to be 130 × BSA in mL/min ($\dot{V}O_2$)

P: Pressure in cm H_2O or mm Hg

Δ*P*:   Pressure change in cm H_2O

$\overline{PA}$:   Mean pulmonary artery pressure in mm Hg

$PA_{systolic}$:   Systolic pulmonary artery pressure in mm Hg

$P_{(A-a)}O_2$:   Alveolar–arterial oxygen tension gradient in mm Hg

P_aCO_2:   Arterial carbon dioxide tension in mm Hg

P_AO_2:   Alveolar oxygen tension in mm Hg

P_aO_2:   Arterial oxygen tension in mm Hg

P_B: Barometric pressure in mm Hg

PCWP: Pulmonary capillary wedge pressure in mm Hg

P_ECO_2:   Mixed expired carbon dioxide tension in mm Hg

PEEP: Positive end-expiratory pressure in cm H_2O

P_g: Partial pressure of a dry gas

pH: Puissance hydrogen, negative logarithm of H^+ ion concentration

P_{H_2O}:   Water vapor pressure, 47 mm Hg saturated at 37°C

PIP: Peak inspiratory pressure in cm H_2O

P_{max} Maximum airway pressure in cm H_2O (peak airway pressure)

psig: Pounds per square inch, a gauge pressure

P_{st}:   Static airway pressure in cm H_2O (plateau airway pressure)

$P_{\bar{v}}O_2$:   Mixed venous oxygen tension in mm Hg

PVR: Pulmonary vascular resistance in dyne·sec/cm^5

$Q_{sp}/\dot{Q}_T$:   Physiologic shunt to total perfusion ratio in %

Q_T: Total perfusion in L/min; cardiac output (CO)

R: Resistance in cm H_2O/L/sec

RA: Right atrial pressure in mm Hg

$\overline{RA}$:   Mean right atrial pressure in mm Hg

R_{aw}:   Airway resistance in cm H_2O/L/sec

RH: Relative humidity in %

RR: Respiratory rate per minute; frequency

$RSBI$:   Rapid Shallow Breathing Index

RV: Residual volume in mL or L

$RVSW$:   Right ventricular stroke work in g·m/beat

$RVSWI$:   Right ventricular stroke work index in g·m/beat/ m^2

S_aO_2:   Arterial oxygen saturation in %

sec: Second

SV: Stroke volume in mL or L

SVI: Stroke volume index in mL/m^2

$S_{\bar{v}}O_2$:   Mixed venous oxygen saturation in vol%

SVR: Systemic vascular resistance in dyne·sec/cm^5

SWI: Simplified Weaning Index

t: Time constant in seconds

TLC: Total lung capacity

torr: Unit of pressure measurement (mm Hg); 1 torr equals 0.1333 kPa

V: (1) Volume in mL or L

      (2) Corrected tidal volume in mL or L

ΔV: Volume change in mL or L

$\dot{V}_A$:   Alveolar minute ventilation in L

VC: Vital capacity in mL or L

V_D: Deadspace volume in mL or L

V_D/V_T: Deadspace to tidal volume ratio in %

$\dot{V}_E$:   Expired minute ventilation in L

$\dot{V}O_2$: O_2 consumption in mL/min

V_T: Tidal volume in mL or L

V_T mech: Mechanical ventilator tidal volume in mL

V_T spon: Patient's spontaneous tidal volume in mL

Vol%:   Volume percent

Volume$_{ATPS}$:   Gas volume saturated with water at ambient (room) temperature and pressure

Volume$_{BTPS}$:   Gas volume saturated with water at body temperature (37°C) and ambient pressure

7

Units of Measurement

Pressure Conversions

cm H$_2$O	mm Hg	psig	kPa
1	0.735	0.0142	0.09806
1.36	1	0.0193	0.1333
70.31	51.7	1	6.895
10.197	7.501	0.145	1

EXAMPLES

To convert cm H$_2$O to mm Hg, multiply cm H$_2$O by 0.735. For example, a central venous pressure reading of 9 cm H$_2$O is about 6.6 mm Hg (9 × 0.735 = 6.615).

To convert mm Hg to cm H$_2$O, multiply mm Hg by 1.36. For example, sea-level barometric pressure of 760 mm Hg is about 1,034 cm H$_2$O (760 × 1.36 = 1033.6).

To convert psig to mm Hg, multiply psig by 51.7. For example, a piped-in oxygen gas source of 50 psig equals 2,585 mm Hg (50 × 51.7 = 2,585).

French (Fr) and Millimeter (mm) Conversions

Millimeter (mm)	French (Fr)
1	3
0.33	1

EXAMPLES

To convert mm to Fr, multiply mm by 3. For example, an endotracheal tube with an internal diameter (*ID*) of 2.5 mm equals 7.5 Fr (2.5 × 3).

To convert Fr to mm, multiply Fr by 0.33 or divide Fr by 3. For example, a 12-Fr suction catheter equals 4 mm (12 × 0.33 or 12/3).

Conversions of Conventional and Système International (SI) Units

MEASUREMENT	CONVENTIONAL UNIT	SI UNIT	CONVERSION FACTOR
Pressure	cm H_2O	kilopascal (kPa)	0.09806
	mm Hg (torr)	kPa	0.1333
	lb/in^2 (psi)	kPa	6.895
Compliance	L/cm H_2O	L/k/Pa	10.20
Resistance	cm H_2O/L/sec	kPa/L/sec	0.09806
Work	kilogram-meter (kg-M)	joule (J)	9.807
Length	inch (in)	meter (m)	0.0254
	foot (ft)	m	0.3048
Area	in^2	cm^2	6.452
Volume	ft^3	liter (L)	28.32

EXAMPLES

To convert a conventional unit to an SI unit, *multiply* the conventional unit by the conversion factor. For example, convert 40 mm Hg to kPa:

40 mm Hg = 40 × 0.1333 = 5.33 kPa.

To convert an SI unit to a conventional unit, *divide* the SI unit by the conversion factor. For example, convert 350 kPa to lb/in^2 (psi):

$$350 \text{ kPa} = \frac{350}{6.895} = 50.76 \text{ psi.}$$

REFERENCE

Pierson

Conversions of Other Units of Measurement

Metric Weight

GRAMS	CENTIGRAMS	MILLIGRAMS	MICROGRAMS	NANOGRAMS
1	100	1,000	1,000,000	1,000,000,000
0.01	1	10	10,000	10,000,000
0.001	0.1	1	1,000	1,000,000
0.000001	0.0001	0.001	1	1,000
0.000000001	0.0000001	0.000001	0.001	1

Metric Liquid

LITER	CENTILITER	MILLILITER	MICROLITER	NANOLITER
1	100	1,000	1,000,000	1,000,000,000
0.01	1	10	10,000	10,000,000
0.001	0.1	1	1,000	1,000,000
0.000001	0.0001	0.001	1	1,000
0.000000001	0.0000001	0.000001	0.001	1

Metric Length

METER	CENTIMETER	MILLIMETER	MICROMETER	NANOMETER
1	100	1,000	1,000,000	1,000,000,000
0.01	1	10	10,000	10,000,000
0.001	0.1	1	1,000	1,000,000
0.000001	0.0001	0.001	1	1,000
0.000000001	0.0000001	0.000001	0.001	1

Weight Conversions (Metric and Avoirdupois)

GRAMS	KILOGRAMS	OUNCES	POUNDS
1	0.001	0.0353	0.0022
1000	1	35.3	2.2
28.41	0.02841	1	$\frac{1}{16}$
454.5	0.4545	16	1

Weight Conversions (Metric and Apothecary)

GRAMS	MILLIGRAMS	GRAINS	DRAMS	OUNCES	POUNDS
1	1,000	15.4	0.2577	0.0322	0.00268
0.001	1	0.0154	0.00026	0.0000322	0.00000268
0.0648	64.8	1	$\frac{1}{60}$	$\frac{1}{480}$	$\frac{1}{5,760}$
3.888	3,888	60	1	$\frac{1}{8}$	$\frac{1}{96}$
31.1	31,104	480	8	1	$\frac{1}{12}$
373.25	373,248	5,760	96	12	1

Weight

METRIC	APPROXIMATE APOTHECARY EQUIVALENTS
Grams	*Grains*
0.0002	$\frac{1}{300}$
0.0003	$\frac{1}{200}$
0.0004	$\frac{1}{150}$
0.0005	$\frac{1}{120}$
0.0006	$\frac{1}{100}$
0.001	$\frac{1}{60}$
0.002	$\frac{1}{30}$
0.005	$\frac{1}{12}$
0.010	$\frac{1}{6}$
0.015	$\frac{1}{4}$
0.025	$\frac{3}{8}$
0.030	$\frac{1}{2}$
0.050	$\frac{3}{4}$
0.060	1
0.100	$1\frac{1}{2}$
0.120	2
0.200	3
0.300	5
0.500	$7\frac{1}{2}$
0.600	10
1	15
2	30
4	60

Liquid Measure

METRIC	APPROXIMATE APOTHECARY EQUIVALENTS
Milliliters	
1,000	1 quart
750	1½ pints
500	1 pint
250	8 fluid ounces
200	7 fluid ounces
100	3½ fluid ounces
50	1¾ fluid ounces
30	1 fluid ounce
15	4 fluid drams
10	2½ fluid drams
8	2 fluid drams
5	1¼ fluid drams
4	1 fluid dram
3	45 minims
2	30 minims
1	15 minims
0.75	12 minims
0.6	10 minims
0.5	8 minims
0.3	5 minims
0.25	4 minims
0.2	3 minims
0.1	1½ minims
0.06	1 minim
0.05	¾ minim
0.03	½ minim

Volume Conversions: (Metric and Apothecary)

MILLILITERS	MINIMS	FLUID DRAMS	FLUID OUNCES	PINTS	LITERS	GALLONS	QUARTS	FLUID OUNCES	PINTS
1	16.2	0.27	0.0338	0.0021	1	0.2642	1.057	33.824	2.114
0.0616	1	1/60	1/480	1/7680	3.785	1	4	128	8
3.697	60	1	⅛	1/128	0.946	¼	1	32	2
29.58	480	8	1	1/16	0.473	⅛	½	16	1
473.2	7,680	128	16	1	0.0296	1/128	1/32	1	1/16

Length Conversions (Metric and English Systems)					
	MILLIMETERS	**CENTIMETERS**	**INCHES**	**FEET**	**YARDS**	**METERS**
1Å =	$\dfrac{1}{10,000,000}$	$\dfrac{1}{100,000,000}$	$\dfrac{1}{254,000,000}$	$\dfrac{1}{3,050,000,000}$	$\dfrac{1}{9,140,000,000}$	$\dfrac{1}{10,000,000,000}$
1 nm =	$\dfrac{1}{1,000,000}$	$\dfrac{1}{10,000,000}$	$\dfrac{1}{25,400,000}$	$\dfrac{1}{305,000,000}$	$\dfrac{1}{914,000,000}$	$\dfrac{1}{1,000,000,000}$
1 μ =	$\dfrac{1}{1000}$	$\dfrac{1}{10,000}$	$\dfrac{1}{25,000}$	$\dfrac{1}{305,000}$	$\dfrac{1}{914,000}$	$\dfrac{1}{1,000,000}$
1 mm =	1.0	0.1	0.03937	0.00328	0.0011	0.001
1 cm =	10.0	1.0	0.3937	0.03281	0.0109	0.01
1 in =	25.4	2.54	1.0	0.0833	0.0278	0.0254
1 ft =	304.8	30.48	12.0	1.0	0.333	0.3048
1 yd =	914.40	91.44	36.0	3.0	1.0	0.9144
1 m =	1000.0	100.0	39.37	3.2808	1.0936	1.0

REFERENCE   Des Jardin

Listing of Appendices

A—Anatomical Values in Children and Adults
B—Apgar Score
C—Barometric Pressures at Selected Altitudes
D—Basal Metabolic Rate
E—Conversion Factors for Duration of Gas Cylinders
F—Conversion Factors from ATPS to BTPS
G—Croup Score
H—Croup Score Modified Westley
I—Dubois Body Surface Chart
J—Electrolyte Concentrations in Plasma
K—Endotracheal Tubes and Suction Catheters
L—Energy Expenditure, Resting and Total
M—Fagerstrom Nicotine Dependence Test for Cigarette Smokers
N—French and Millimeter Conversion
O—Glasgow Coma Score
P—Harris Benedict Formula
Q—Hemodynamic Normal Ranges
R—Humidity Capacity of Saturated Gas at Selected Temperatures
S—Logarithm Table
T—Lung Volumes, Capacities, and Ventilation
U—Neonatal Blood Pressure
V—Oxygen Transport
W—Reference Laboratory Values
X—P_AO_2 at Selected F_IO_2
Y—Partial Pressure (in mm Hg) of Gases in the Air, Alveoli, and Blood
Z—Periodic Chart of Elements
AA—Pitting Edema Scale
BB—Pressure Conversions
CC—Ramsay Sedation Scale
DD—Revised Sedation Scale
EE—Richmond Agitation and Sedation Scale
FF—Sedation Agitation Scale
GG—Therapeutic Blood Levels of Selected Drugs
HH—Weaning Criteria

A
Anatomical Values in Children and Adults

Age	Weight		Height		BSA	Tracheal length		Tracheal diameter	
	Kg	lb	cm	ft/in	m^2	cm	in	mm	in
Newborn	3.4	7.5	50	19.7″	0.2	4.0	1.57	3.8	0.15
3 months	5	11	60	2′1″	0.33	4.2	1.65	4.8	0.19
6 months	7.5	17	66	2′2″	0.38	4.2	1.65	5.6	0.22
1 year	10.0	22	75	2′6″	0.47	4.5	1.77	6.5	0.26
1.5 years	11.4	25	82	2′8″	0.52	4.5	1.77	6.5–7.0	0.26–0.28
2 years	12.5	28	86	2′10″	0.56	5.0	1.97	7.0	0.28
3 years	13–15	31	96	3′2″	0.62	5.3	2.09	8.0	0.32
4 years	16.5	36	103	3′5″	0.68	5.4	2.13	8.0	0.32
5 years	18.4	41	109	3′7″	0.75	5.6	2.21	8.0–9.0	0.32–0.35
6 years	22.0	48	117	3′10″	0.85	5.7	2.24	9.0	0.35
8 years	27.3	60	124	4′1″	0.92	6.0	2.36	9.0	0.35
10 years	32.6	72	140	4′7″	1.12	6.3	2.48	9–11	0.35–0.43
14 years	49.0	108	163	5′4″	1.50	6.4	2.53	11–15	0.43–0.59
Adult	60–80	132–176	172	5′8″	1.7–1.9	10–12	3.9–4.7	13–25	0.51–0.98

Adapted from: Noack, G. (1993). *Ventilatory Treatment of Neonates and Infants.* Solna, Sweden: Siemens-Elema AB Life Support Systems Division, Marketing Communications.

B

Apgar Score

Normal: 7 to 10 at 1-minute and 5-minute after birth

Test	0 Points	1 Point	2 Points
Activity (Muscle Tone)	Absent	Arms and legs extended	Active movement with flexed arms and legs
Pulse (Heart Rate)	Absent	Below 100 bpm	Above 100 bpm
Grimace (Response Stimulation or Reflex Irritability)	No Response	Facial grimace	Sneeze, cough, pulls away
Appearance (Skin Color)	Blue-gray, pale all over	Pink body and blue extremities	Normal over entire body; completely pink
Respiration (Breathing)	Absent	Slow, irregular	Good, crying

The APGAR score is checked at 1 minute after birth, 5 minutes after birth, and if indicated, every 5 minutes thereafter. This scoring system is used strictly to determine the neonate's immediate condition at birth and does not reflect the future condition of the neonate.

MANAGEMENT STRATEGIES

- Apgar 7–10 (normal)—Suction with bulb syringe; keep dry and warm (skin to skin with mother and blanket).
- Apgar 4–6: Suction with bulb syringe; ventilate 40–60 breaths/min with 100% oxygen; monitor heart rate; begin cardiac compressions if heart rate not increasing after 15–30 seconds of assisted ventilations; keep warm and dry.
- Apgar 0–3: Suction with bulb syringe; support ventilation 40–60 breath/min with 100% oxygen, bag and mask, intubate if bagging inadequate; monitor; if heart rate < 80/min and not increasing with assisted ventilation after 15–30 seconds, begin cardiac compression; keep warm and dry.

REFERENCES

childbirth.org/articles/apgar.html
sonoma-county.org/cvrems/resources/pdf/guidelines/9405.pdf

C

Barometric Pressures at Selected Altitudes

	Feet	Meters	P_B (mm Hg)
Below sea level	−66	−20	2,280
	−33	−10	1,520
Sea level	0	0	760
Above sea level	2,000	610	707
	4,000	1,219	656
	6,000[a]	1,829	609
	8,000	2,438	564
	10,000	3,048	523
	12,000	3,658	483
	14,000[b]	4,267	446
	16,000	4,877	412
	18,000	5,486	379
	20,000	6,096	349
	22,000	6,706	321
	24,000	7,315	294
	26,000	7,925	270
	28,000	8,534	247
	30,000[c]	9,144	226
	32,000	9,754	206
	34,000	10,363	187
	36,000	10,973	170
	40,000	12,192	141
	50,000	15,240	87
	63,000	19,202	47

[a] Denver, Colorado, 5,280 ft
[b] Mount Elbert, Colorado, 14,433 ft
[c] Mount Everest, 29,028 ft

D

Basal Metabolic Rate

The Basal Metabolic Rate (BMD) is used in the Harris Benedict Equation to calculate daily calorie needs based on a person's activity level.

ENGLISH BMR FORMULA

- Women: BMR = 655 + (4.35 × weight in pounds) + (4.7 × height in inches) − (4.7 × age in years)
- Men: BMR = 66 + (6.23 × weight in pounds) + (12.7 × height in inches) − (6.8 × age in years)

METRIC BMR FORMULA

- Women: BMR = 655 + (9.6 × weight in kilos) + (1.85 × height in cm) − (4.7 × age in years)
- Men: BMR = 66 + (13.7 × weight in kilos) + (5 × height in cm) − (6.8 × age in years)

REFERENCE

calculatorslive.com/BMR-Calculator.aspx

E
Conversion Factors for Duration of Gas Cylinders

Cylinder Size	B/BB	D/DD	E	M	G	H/K
Carbon Dioxide (CO_2)	0.17	0.43	0.72	3.44	5.59	7.18
Carbon Dioxide/Oxygen (CO_2/O_2)		0.18	0.3	1.36	2.42	2.73
Cyclopropane (C_3H_6)	0.17	0.40				
Helium (He)		0.14	0.23	1.03	1.82	2.73
Helium/Oxygen (He/O_2)			0.23	1.03	1.82	2.05
Nitrous Oxide (N_2O)		0.43	0.72	3.44	6.27	7.18
Oxygen (O_2)	0.09	0.18	0.28	1.57	2.41	3.14
Air (N_2/O_2)		0.17	0.28	1.49	2.30	2.98
Nitrogen (N_2)			0.28			2.91

(Conversion factors are based on full cylinder at pressure of 2,200 psig.)
To calculate duration of gas cylinder at a constant liter flow: (1) multiply the conversion factor by the pressure reading on the gas gauge; (2) divide the product from (1) by the liter flow in use; (3) answer equals the duration, in minutes, of gas cylinder at the same liter flow.

$$\text{Duration} = \frac{\text{Conversion factor} \times \text{Psig}}{\text{Liter flow}}$$

For example, see Oxygen Duration of E Cylinder and Oxygen Duration of H or K Cylinder.

F

Conversion Factors from ATPS to BTPS

Gas Temperature (°C)	Factors to Convert to 37°C Saturated*	Water Vapor Pressure (mm Hg)
18	1.112	15.6
19	1.107	16.5
20	1.102	17.5
21	1.096	18.7
22	1.091	19.8
23	1.085	21.1
24	1.080	22.4
25	1.075	23.8
26	1.068	25.2
27	1.063	26.7
28	1.057	28.3
29	1.051	30.0
30	1.045	31.8
31	1.039	33.7
32	1.032	35.7
33	1.026	37.7
34	1.020	39.9
35	1.014	42.2
36	1.007	44.6
37	1.000	47.0
38	0.993	49.8
39	0.986	52.5
40	0.979	55.4
41	0.971	58.4
42	0.964	61.6

*Conversion factors are based on P_B = 760 mm Hg. For other barometric pressures and temperatures, use the following equation: $Conversion\ factor = \dfrac{P_B - P_{H_2O}}{P_B - 47} \times \dfrac{310}{(273 + °C)}$

G
Croup Score

INTERPRETATION

≤4 mild croup
5 to 6 mild/moderate croup
7 to 8 moderate croup
≥9 severe croup

Clinical Indicator	Score
Inspiratory Stridor	
None	0
When agitated	1
Intermittent at rest	2
Continuous at rest	3
Retractions	
None	0
Mild	1
Moderate	2
Severe	3
Air Movement	
Normal	0
Decreased	1
Moderately decreased	2
Severely decreased	3
Cyanosis	
None	0
Dusky	1
Cyanotic on room air	2
Cyanotic with supplemental oxygen	3
Level of Alertness	
Alert (0 points)	0
Restless or anxious (1 points)	1
Lethargic/Obtunded (2 points)	2

REFERENCE

pediatrics.about.com/cs/commoninfectons/a/croup.htm

H
Croup Score
Modified Westley

INTERPRETATION

>8 indicates respiratory failure

Clinical Indicator	Score
Inspiratory stridor	
None	0
At rest, with stethoscope	1
At rest, no stethoscope required to hear	2
Level of consciousness	
Normal	0
Altered	5
Air entry	
Normal	0
Decreased	1
Severe decreased	2
Cyanosis	
None	0
Agitated	4
Resting	5
Retractions	
None	0
Mild	1
Moderate	2
Severe	3

REFERENCES

Bjornson, C. L., et al. (1992). *N Engl J Med, 351,* 1306–1313.
Geelhoed, G. C. (2004). *Pediatr Pulmonol, 20:6,* 362–368.
Klassen, T. P. (1998). *JAMA, 279:20,* 1629–1632.
Rittichier, K. K. (2000). *Pediatrics, 106(6),* 1344–1348.
Waisman, Y. (1992). *Pediatrics, 89:2,* 302–306.

I
DuBois Body Surface Chart

Directions

To find body surface of a patient, locate the height in inches (or centimeters) on Scale I and the weight in pounds (or kilograms) on Scale II and place a straight edge (ruler) between these two points, which will intersect Scale III at the patient's surface area.

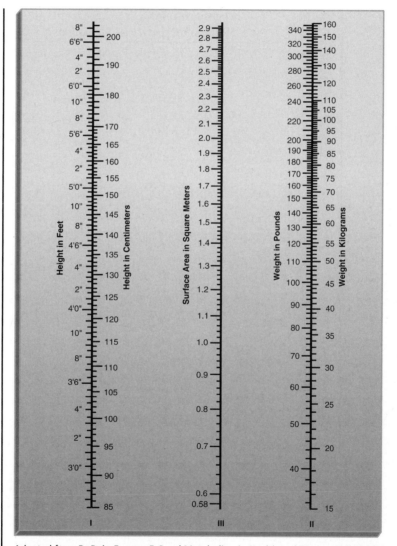

Adapted from DuBois, Eugene F. *Basal Metabolism in Health and Disease*. Philadelphia: Lea and Febiger, 1924.

Source: Des Jardin, T.R. *Cardiopulmonary Anatomy and Physiology: Essentials for Respiratory Care*, 5th ed. Clifton Park, NY: Delmar Cengage Learning, 2008.

J
Electrolyte Concentrations in Plasma

Cations	Concentration (Range) mEq/L	Anions	Concentration (Range) mEq/L
Na^+	140 (138 to 142)	Cl^-	103 (101 to 105)
K^+	4 (3 to 5)	HCO_3^-	25 (23 to 27)
Ca^{++}	5 (4.5 to 5.5)	Protein	16 (14 to 18)
Mg^{++}	2 (1.5 to 2.5)	HPO_4^{--}, $H_2PO_4^-$	2 (1.5 to 2.5)
Total	151	SO_4^{--}	1 (0.8 to 1.2)
		Organic acids	4 (3.5 to 4.5)
		Total	151

K
Endotracheal Tubes and Suction Catheters

Age	Weight (g/Kg)	Internal Diameter (ID) (mm)	Oral Length* (cm)	Suction Catheter (French)
Newborn (<28 weeks)	<1000 g	2.5	7	5 or 6
Newborn (28–34 weeks)	1000–2000 g	3.0	8	6 or 8
Newborn (34–38 weeks)	2000–3000 g	3.5	9	8
Newborn (>38 weeks)	>3000 g	3.5–4.0	10	8 for 3.5 mm
				10 for 4.0 mm
Infant under 6 months		3.5–4.0	10	8
Infant under 1 year		4.0–4.5	11	8
Child under 2 years		4.5–5.0	12	8
Child over 2 years		(Age/4) + 4	(Age/2) + 12	10
Adult female		7.0–8.0	20–22	12
Adult male		8.0–8.5	20–22	14

Notes: Use uncuffed ET tube for children under age 8 years (normal narrowing at cricoids serves as natural cuff).
*ET tube with one marking at bottom of tube: the marking should be at vocal cord level.
ET tube with two markings at bottom of tube: the vocal cords should be between these two markings.

REFERENCE

fpnotebook.com/lung/Procedure/EndtrchlTb.htm

L
Energy Expenditure, Resting and Total

CALCULATION OF RESTING ENERGY EXPENDITURE (REE)

REE for men in kcal/day = 66 + (13.7 × kg) + (5.0 × cm) − (6.8 × years)

REE for women in kcal/day = 655 + (9.6 × kg) + (1.85 × cm) − (4.7 × years)

CALCULATION OF TOTAL ENERGY EXPENDITURE (TEE)

TEE for men in kcal/day = REE × Activity Factor × Stress Factor

TEE for women in kcal/day = REE × Activity Factor × Stress Factor

Activity Factor
    Confined to bed × 1.2
    Out of bed × 1.3

Stress Factor
    Minor operation × 1.20
    Skeletal trauma × 1.35
    Major sepsis × 1.60
    Severe thermal burn × 2.10

M
Fagerstrom Nicotine Dependence Test for Cigarette Smokers

1. How soon after you wake up do you smoke your first cigarette?
   Within 5 minutes (3 points) _____
   5 to 30 minutes (2 points) _____
   31 to 60 minutes (1 point) _____
   After 60 minutes (0 points) _____

2. Do you find it difficult not to smoke in places where smoking is prohibited?
   Yes (1 point) _____
   No (0 points) _____

3. Which cigarette would you most hate to give up?
   The first one in the morning (1 point) _____
   Any other one (0 points) _____

4. How many cigarettes do you smoke each day?
   31 or more (3 points) _____
   21 to 30 (2 points) _____
   11 to 20 (1 point) _____
   10 or fewer (0 points) _____

5. Do you smoke more during the first few hours after waking up than during the rest of the day?
   Yes (1 point) _____
   No (0 points) _____

6. Do you still smoke if you are so sick that you are in bed most of the day, or if you have a cold or the flu and have trouble breathing?
   Yes (1 point) _____
   No (0 points) _____

Scoring	Nicotine Dependence
0	No dependence
1–2	Low dependence
3–5	Moderately dependent
6–8	Highly dependent
9–10	Very dependent

REFERENCE

nova.edu/gsc/nicotine_risk.html

N

French and Millimeter Conversions

Millimeter (mm)	French (Fr)
1	3
0.33	1

O

Glasgow Coma Score

Glasgow coma score (GCS)* ranges from 3 to 15 and is composed of three parameters: best eye response, best verbal response, and best motor response. The GCS is typically reported in its components such as E2V1M3 5 GCS 6. A GCS score of 13 to 14 correlates with a mild brain injury, 9 to 12 suggests a moderate injury, and 8 or less a severe brain injury.

BEST EYE RESPONSE (1 TO 4)

1. No eye opening
2. Eye opening to pain
3. Eye opening to verbal command
4. Eyes open spontaneously

BEST VERBAL RESPONSE (1 TO 5)

1. No verbal response
2. Incomprehensible sounds
3. Inappropriate words
4. Confused
5. Orientated

BEST MOTOR RESPONSE (1 TO 6)

1. No motor response
2. Extension to pain
3. Flexion to pain
4. Withdrawal from pain
5. Localizing pain
6. Obeys Commands

REFERENCE

Teasdale, G. and Jennett, B. (1974). "Assessment of coma and impaired consciousness: A practical scale," *The Lancet, 304,* 81–84.

P

Harris Benedict Formula

To determine the total daily calorie needs, multiply Harris Benedict Formula (BMR) by the appropriate activity factor:

- Sedentary (little or no exercise): Calories = BMR × 1.2
- Lightly active (light exercise/sports 1–3 days/week): Calories = BMR × 1.375
- Moderately active (moderate exercise/sports 3–5 days/week): Calories = BMR × 1.55
- Very active (hard exercise/sports 6–7 days a week): Calories = BMR × 1.725
- Extra active (very hard exercise/sports and physical job or 2x training): Calories = BMR × 1.9

REFERENCE

bmi-calculator.net/bmr-calculator/harris-benedict-equation/

Q

Hemodynamic Normal Ranges

Hemodynamic Values Directly Obtained by Pulmonary Artery Catheter

Hemodynamic Value	Abbreviation	Normal Range
Central venous pressure	CVP	1 to 7 mm Hg
Right atrial pressure	RAP	1 to 7 mm Hg
Mean pulmonary artery pressure	$\overline{PA}$	15 mm Hg
Pulmonary capillary wedge pressure	PCWP	8 to 12 mm Hg
(also called pulmonary artery wedge pressure;	PAWP	
pulmonary artery occlusion pressure)	PAOP	
Cardiac output	CO	4 to 8 L/min

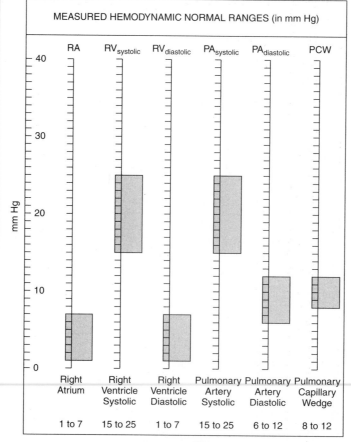

MEASURED HEMODYNAMIC NORMAL RANGES (in mm Hg)

	RA	RV$_{systolic}$	RV$_{diastolic}$	PA$_{systolic}$	PA$_{diastolic}$	PCW
	Right Atrium	Right Ventricle Systolic	Right Ventricle Diastolic	Pulmonary Artery Systolic	Pulmonary Artery Diastolic	Pulmonary Capillary Wedge
	1 to 7	15 to 25	1 to 7	15 to 25	6 to 12	8 to 12

mm Hg

Adapted from Des Jardins, T.R. *Cardiopulmonary Anatomy and Physiology: Essentials for Respiratory Care*, 5th ed. Clifton Park, NY: Delmar Cengage Learning, 2008.

Computed Hemodynamic Values:

Hemodynamic Variable	Abbreviation	Normal Range
Stroke volume	SV	40 to 80 mL
Stroke volume index	SVI	33 to 47 L/beat/m^2
Cardiac index	CI	2.5 to 3.5 L/min/m^2
Right ventricular stroke work index	RVSWI	7 to 12 g·m/beat/m^2
Left ventricular stroke work index	LVSWI	40 to 60 g·m/beat/m^2
Pulmonary vascular resistance	PVR	50 to 150 dyne·sec/cm^5
Systemic vascular resistance	SVR	800 to 1500 dyne·sec/cm^5

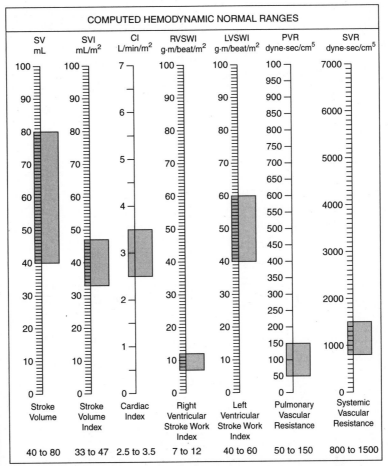

Modified from Des Jardins, T.R. *Cardiopulmonary Anatomy and Physiology: Essentials for Respiratory Care,* 5th ed. Clifton Park, NY: Delmar Cengage Learning, 2008.

R

Humidity Capacity of Saturated Gas at Selected Temperatures

Gas Temperature (°C)	Water Content (mg/L)	Water Vapor Pressure (mm Hg)
0	4.9	4.6
5	6.8	6.6
10	9.4	9.3
17	14.5	14.6
18	15.4	15.6
19	16.3	16.5
20	17.3	17.5
21	18.4	18.7
22	19.4	19.8
23	20.6	21.1
24	21.8	22.4
25	23.1	23.8
26	24.4	25.2
27	25.8	26.7
28	27.2	28.3
29	28.8	30.0
30	30.4	31.8
31	32.0	33.7
32	33.8	35.7
33	35.6	37.7
34	37.6	39.9
35	39.6	42.2
36	41.7	44.6
37	43.9	47.0
38	46.2	49.8
39	48.6	52.5
40	51.1	55.4
41	53.7	58.4
42	56.5	61.6
43	59.5	64.9

S

Logarithm Table

TERMINOLOGY

$\log 20 = 1.301$

$\downarrow \quad \downarrow \quad \downarrow \downarrow$

a   b   c d

a: logarithm, b: number, c: characteristic, d: mantissa.

EXAMPLE 1

Find the logarithm for 30.4.

Step 1. From the log table find the number 30 along the vertical column (N).
Step 2. Find the number 4 along the horizontal row (N).
Step 3. The mantissa intersected by the column and row should read 4829.
Step 4. Since the number 30.4 has two digits in front of the decimal point, use 1. in front of the mantissa.
Log 30.4 becomes 1.4829.

NOTE

The characteristic is determined by the number of digits in front of the decimal point. The characteristic is 0. for one digit in front of the decimal point; 1. for two digits; 2. for three digits; and so on.
For example, the answer for log 304 is 2.4829. You may notice that the mantissa for 304 is same as that for 30.4 and that the only change is in the characteristic. The following examples should clarify this point:

$\log 0.0304 = \overline{2}.4829$
$\log 0.304 = \overline{1}.4829$
$\log 3.04 = 0.4829$
$\log 30.4 = 1.4829$
$\log 304 = 2.4829$
$\log 3040 = 3.4829$

EXAMPLE 2

Find the logarithms for 18.7 and 187.

Step 1. From the log table find the number 18 along the vertical column (N).
Step 2. Find the number 7 along the horizontal row (N).
Step 3. The mantissa intersected by the column and row should read 2718.
Step 4. Because the number 18.7 has two digits in front of the decimal point, use 1. in front of the mantissa. Log 18.7 becomes 1.2718. Because the number 187 has three digits in front of the decimal point, use 2. in front of the mantissa. Log 187 becomes 2.2718.

EXERCISE 1   Find the logarithm for 22.2.

[Answer: log 22.2 = 1.3464]

EXERCISE 2   Find the logarithm for 30.15.

[Answer: log 30.15 = 1.4793. Look for the mantissas under 1 and 2 and find the average.]

Common Logarithms of Numbers[a]

N	0	1	2	3	4	5	6	7	8	9
10	0000	0043	0086	0128	0170	0212	0253	0294	0334	0374
11	0414	0453	0492	0531	0569	0607	0645	0682	0719	0755
12	0792	0828	0864	0899	0934	0969	1004	1038	1072	1106
13	1139	1173	1206	1239	1271	1303	1335	1367	1399	1430
14	1461	1492	1523	1553	1584	1614	1644	1673	1703	1732
15	1761	1790	1818	1847	1875	1903	1931	1959	1987	2014
16	2041	2068	2095	2122	2148	2175	2201	2227	2253	2279
17	2304	2330	2335	2380	2405	2430	2455	2480	2504	2529
18	2553	2577	2601	2625	2648	2672	2695	2718	2742	2765
19	2788	2810	2833	2856	2878	2900	2923	2945	2967	2989
20	3010	3032	3054	3075	3096	3118	3139	3160	3181	3201
21	3222	3243	3263	3284	3304	3324	3345	3365	3385	3404
22	3424	3444	3464	3483	3502	3522	3541	3560	3579	3598
23	3617	3636	3655	3674	3692	3711	3729	3747	3766	3784
24	3802	3820	3838	3856	3874	3892	3909	3927	3945	3962
25	3979	3997	4014	4031	4048	4065	4082	4099	4116	4133
26	4150	4166	4183	4200	4216	4232	4249	4265	4281	4298
27	4314	4330	4346	4362	4378	4393	4409	4425	4440	4456
28	4472	4487	4502	4518	4533	4548	4564	4579	4594	4609
29	4624	4639	4654	4669	4683	4698	4713	4728	4742	4757
30	4771	4786	4800	4814	4829	4843	4857	4871	4886	4900
31	4914	4928	4942	4955	4969	4983	4997	5011	5024	5038
32	5051	5065	5079	5092	5105	5119	5132	5145	5159	5172
33	5185	5198	5211	5224	5237	5250	5263	5276	5289	5302
34	5315	5328	5340	5353	5366	5378	5391	5403	5416	5428
35	5441	5453	5465	5478	5490	5502	5514	5527	5539	5551
36	5563	5575	5587	5599	5611	5623	5635	5647	5658	5670
37	5682	5694	5705	5717	5729	5740	5752	5763	5775	5786
38	5798	5809	5821	5832	5843	5855	5866	5877	5888	5899
39	5911	5922	5933	5944	5955	5966	5977	5988	5999	6010
40	6021	6031	6042	6053	6064	6075	6085	6096	6107	6117
41	6128	6138	6149	6160	6170	6180	6191	6201	6212	6222
42	6232	6243	6253	6263	6274	6284	6294	6304	6314	6325
43	6335	6345	6355	6365	6375	6385	6395	6405	6415	6425
44	6435	6444	6454	6464	6474	6484	6493	6503	6513	6522
45	6532	6542	6551	6561	6571	6580	6590	6599	6609	6618
46	6628	6637	6646	6656	6665	6675	6684	6693	6702	6712
47	6721	6730	6739	6749	6758	6767	6776	6785	6794	6803
48	6812	6821	6830	6839	6848	6857	6866	6875	6884	6893
49	6902	6911	6920	6928	6937	6946	6955	6964	6972	6981
50	6990	6998	7007	7016	7024	7033	7042	7050	7059	7067
51	7076	7084	7093	7101	7110	7118	7126	7135	7143	7152
52	7160	7168	7177	7185	7193	7202	7210	7218	7226	7235
53	7243	7251	7259	7267	7275	7284	7292	7300	7308	7316
54	7324	7332	7340	7348	7356	7364	7372	7380	7388	7396

N	0	1	2	3	4	5	6	7	8	9
55	7404	7412	7419	7427	7435	7443	7451	7459	7466	7474
56	7482	7490	7497	7505	7513	7520	7528	7536	7543	7551
57	7559	7566	7574	7582	7589	7597	7604	7612	7619	7627
58	7634	7642	7649	7657	7664	7672	7679	7686	7694	7701
59	7709	7716	7723	7731	7738	7745	7752	7760	7767	7774
60	7782	7789	7796	7803	7810	7818	7825	7832	7839	7846
61	7853	7860	7868	7875	7892	7889	7896	7903	7910	7917
62	7924	7931	7938	7945	7952	7959	7966	7973	7980	7987
63	7993	8000	8007	8014	8021	8028	8035	8041	8048	8055
64	8062	8069	8075	8082	8089	8096	8102	8109	8116	8122
65	8129	8136	8142	8149	8156	8162	8169	8176	8182	8189
66	8195	8202	8209	8215	8222	8228	8235	8241	8248	8254
67	8261	8267	8274	8280	8287	8293	8299	8306	8312	8319
68	8325	8331	8338	8344	8351	8357	8363	8370	8376	8382
69	8388	8395	8401	8407	8414	8420	8426	8432	8439	8445
70	8451	8457	8463	8470	8476	8482	8488	8494	8500	8506
71	8513	8519	8525	8531	8537	8543	8549	8555	8561	8567
72	8573	8579	8585	8591	8597	8603	8609	8615	8621	8627
73	8633	8639	8645	8651	8657	8663	8669	8675	8681	8686
74	8692	8698	8704	8710	8716	8722	8727	8733	8739	8745
75	8751	8756	8762	8768	8774	8779	8785	8791	8797	8802
76	8808	8814	8820	8825	8831	8837	8842	8848	8854	8859
77	8865	8871	8876	8882	8887	8893	8899	8904	8910	8915
78	8921	8927	8932	8938	8943	8949	8954	8960	8965	8971
79	8976	8982	8987	8993	8998	9004	9009	9015	9020	9025
80	9031	9036	9042	9047	9053	9058	9063	9069	9074	9079
81	9085	9090	9096	9101	9106	9112	9117	9122	9128	9133
82	9138	9143	9149	9154	9159	9165	9170	9175	9180	9186
83	9191	9196	9201	9206	9212	9217	9222	9227	9232	9238
84	9243	9248	9253	9258	9263	9269	9274	9279	9284	9289
85	9294	9299	9304	9309	9315	9320	9325	9330	9335	9340
86	9345	9350	9355	9360	9365	9370	9375	9380	9385	9390
87	9395	9400	9405	9410	9415	9420	9425	9430	9435	9440
88	9445	9450	9455	9460	9465	9469	9474	9479	9484	9489
89	9494	9499	9504	9509	9513	9518	9523	9528	9533	9538
90	9542	9547	9552	9557	9562	9566	9571	9576	9581	9586
91	9590	9595	9600	9605	9609	9614	9619	9624	9628	9633
92	9638	9643	9647	9652	9657	9661	9666	9671	9675	9680
93	9685	9689	9694	9699	9703	9708	9713	9714	9722	9727
94	9731	9736	9741	9745	9750	9754	9759	9763	9768	9773
95	9777	9782	9786	9791	9795	9800	9805	9809	9814	9818
96	9823	9827	9832	9836	9841	9845	9850	9854	9859	9863
97	9868	9872	9877	9881	9886	9890	9894	9899	9903	9908
98	9912	9917	9921	9926	9930	9934	9939	9943	9948	9952
99	9956	9961	9965	9969	9974	9978	9983	9987	9991	9996

[a] This table gives the mantissas of numbers with the decimal point omitted in each case. Characteristics are determined by inspection from the numbers. From Wojciechowski, W.V. Respiratory Care Sciences: An Integrated Approach, 4th ed. Clifton Park, NY: Delmar Cengage Learning 2006.

T

Lung Volumes, Capacities, and Ventilation

Volume	Newborn Infant	Young Adult Male	Approx % of TLC (Young Adult Male)
V_T (mL)	15	500	8 to 10
IRV (mL)	60	3100	50
ERV (mL)	40	1200	20
RV (mL)	40	1200	20
IC (mL)	75	3600	60
FRC (mL)	80	2400	40
VC (mL)	115	4800	80
TLC (mL)	155	6000	100
f (bpm)	35 to 50	12 to 20	
$\dot{V}_E$	525 to 750 mL/min	6 to 10 L/min	

Modified from Madama, V.C. *Pulmonary Function Testing and Cardiopulmonary Stress Testing*, 2nd ed. Clifton Park, NY: Delmar Cengage Learning 1998.

REFERENCE

White

U
Neonatal Blood Pressure

Low Birthweight Infants:

Birthweight (g)	Systolic range (mm Hg)	Diastolic range (mm Hg)
501–750	50–62	26–36
751–1000	48–59	23–36
1001–1250	49–61	26–35
1251–1500	46–56	23–33
1501–1750	46–58	23–33
1751–2000	48–61	24–35

Preterm Infants:

Gestation (wk)	Systolic range (mm Hg)	Diastolic range (mm Hg)
<24	48–63	24–39
24–28	48–58	22–36
29–32	47–59	24–34
>32	48–60	24–34

Preterm Infants:

Day	Systolic range (mm Hg)	Diastolic range (mm Hg)
1	48–63	25–35
2	54–63	30–39
3	53–67	31–43
4	57–71	32–45
5	56–72	33–47
6	57–71	32–47
7	61–74	34–46

Term Infants:

Age	Systolic (mm Hg)	Diastolic (mm Hg)	Mean (mm Hg)
1 hour	70	44	53
12 hour	66	41	50
Day 1 (Asleep)	70±9	42±2	55±11
Day 1 (Awake)	71±9	43±10	55±9
Day 3 (Asleep)	75±11	48±10	59±9
Day 3 (Awake)	77±12	49±10	63±13
Day 6 (Asleep)	76±10	46±12	58±12
Day 6 (Awake)	76±10	49±11	62±12
Week 2	78±10	50±9	
Week 3	79±8	49±8	
Week 4	85±10	46±9	

REFERENCE

rch.org.au/nets/handbook/index.cfm?doc_id=450

V

Oxygen Transport

SHADED AREAS REPRESENT NORMAL RANGES

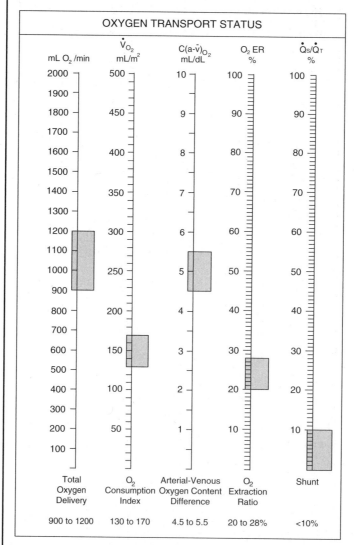

From Des Jardins, T.R. *Cardiopulmonary Anatomy and Physiology: Essentials for Respiratory Care,* 5th ed. Clifton Park, NY: Delmar Cengage Learning, 2008.

W

Reference Laboratory Values

Reference Values for Hematology

Laboratory Tests	Conventional Units	SI Units
Acid hemolysis	No hemolysis	No hemolysis
Alkaline phosphatase	14–100	14–100
Cell counts		
Erythrocytes		
Male	4.6–6.2 million/mm^3	$4.6–6.2 \times 10^{12}$/L
Female	4.2–5.4 million/mm^3	$4.2–5.4 \times 10^{12}$/L
Children (varies with age)	4.5–5.1 million/mm^3	$4.5–5.1 \times 10^{12}$/L
Leukocytes, total	4,500–11,000 million/mm^3	$4.5–11.0 \times 10^{12}$/L
Leukocytes, differential counts		
Myelocytes	0%	0/L
Band neutrophils	3–5%	$150–400 \times 10^{6}$/L
Segmented neutrophils	54–62%	$3,000–5,800 \times 10^{6}$/L
Lymphocytes	25–33%	$1,500–3,000 \times 10^{6}$/L
Monocytes	3–7%	$300–500 \times 10^{6}$/L
Eosinophils	1–3%	$50–250 \times 10^{6}$/L
Basophils	0–1%	$15–50 \times 10^{6}$/L
Platelets	150,000–400,000/mm^3	$150–400 \times 10^{9}$/L
Reticulocytes	25,000–75,000/mm^3	$25–75 \times 10^{9}$/L
Coagulation tests	35–45 sec	
Activated Partial Thromboplastin Time (APTT)		
Bleeding time	2.75–8.0 min	2.75–8.0 min
Coagulation time	5–15 min	5–15 min
D-dimer	<0.5 mcg/mL	<0.5 mg/L
Factor VIII and other coagulation factors	50–150% of normal	0.5–1.5 of normal
Fibrin split products	<10 mcg/mL	<10 mg/L
Fibrinogen	200–400 mg/dL	2.0–4.0 g/L
Partial thromboplastin time (PTT)	20–35 sec	20–35 sec
Prothrombin time/ International Normalized Ratio (INR)	12.0–14.0 sec	12.0–14.0 sec

Laboratory Tests	Conventional Units	SI Units
Coombs' test		
Direct	Negative	
Indirect	Negative	
Corpuscular values of erythrocytes		
Mean corpuscular hemoglobin	26–34 pg/cell	26–34 pg/cell
Mean corpuscular volume	80–96 μm^3	80–96 fL
Mean corpuscular hemoglobin concentration (MCHC)	32–36 g/dL	320–360 g/L
Haptoglobin	20–165 mg/dL	0.20–1.65 g/L
Hematocrit		
Male	40–54 mL/dL	0.40–0.54
Female	37–47 mL/dL	0.37–0.47
Newborn	49–54 ml/dL	0.49–0.54
Children (varies with age)	35–49 ml/dL	0.35–0.49
Hemoglobin		
Male	13.0–18.0 g/dL	8.1–11.2 mmol/L
Female	12.0–16.0 g/dL	7.4–9.9 mmol/L
Newborn	16.5–19.5 g/dL	10.2–12.1 mmol/L
Children (varies with age)	11.2–16.5 g/dL	7.0–10.2 mmol/L
Hemoglobin, fetal	<1.0% of total	<0.01 of total
Hemoglobin A1C	3–5% of total	0.03–0.05 of total
Hemoglobin A2	1.5–3.0% of total	0.015–0.03 of total
Hemoglobin, plasma	0.0–5.0 mg/dL	0.0–3.2 $\mu mol/L$
Methemoglobin	30–130 mg/dL	19–80 $\mu mol/L$
Erythrocyte sedimentation rate (ESR)		
Wintrobe		
Male	0–5 mm/hr	0–5 mm/h
Female	0–15 mm/hr	0–15 mm/h
Westergren		
Male	0–15 mm/hr	0–15 mm/h
Female	0–20 mm/hr	0–20 mm/h

X
P_AO_2 at Selected F_IO_2

F_IO_2*	Calculated P_AO_2**
21%	100
25%	128
30%	164
35%	200
40%	235
45%	271
50%	307
55%	342
60%	388
65%	423
70%	459
75%	495
80%	530
85%	566
90%	602
95%	637
100%	673

* At F_IO_2 of 60% or higher, the factor 1.25 in the equation is omitted.
** The calculated P_AO_2 is based on a PCO_2 of 40 mm Hg, saturated at 37°C, P_B of 760 mm Hg.
$P_AO_2 = (P_B - 47) \times F_IO_2 - (PCO_2 \times 1.25)$.

Y

Partial Pressure (in mm Hg) of Gases in the Air, Alveoli, and Blood*

Gases	Dry Air	Alveolar Gas	Arterial Blood	Venous Blood
P_{O_2}	159.0	100.0	95.0	40.0
P_{CO_2}	0.2	40.0	40.0	46.0
P_{H_2O} (water vapor)	0.0	47.0	47.0	47.0
P_{N_2} (and other gases in minute quantities)	600.8	573.0	573.0	573.0
Total	760.0	760.0	755.0	706.0

* The values shown are based upon standard pressure and temperature.
From Des Jardins, T.R. *Cardiopulmonary Anatomy and Physiology: Essentials for Respiratory Care,* 5th ed. Clifton Park, NY: Delmar Cengage Learning, 2008.

Z
Periodic Chart of Elements

PERIODIC TABLE OF THE ELEMENTS

1 H 1.0079 Hydrogen		
3 Li 1.941 Lithium	4 Be 9.0122 Beryllium	
11 Na 22.990 Sodium	12 Mg 24.305 Magnesium	
19 K 39.098 Potassium	20 Ca 40.078 Calcium	21 Sc 44.956 Scandium
37 Rb 85.468 Rubidium	38 Si 87.62 Strontium	39 Y 88.906 Yttrium
55 Sc 132.91 Caesium	56 Ba 137.33 Barium	57-71 La-Lu
87 Fr 223 Francium	88 Ra 226 Radium	89-103 Ac-Lr

22 Ti 47.867 Titanium; 23 V 50.942 Vanadium; 24 Cr 51.996 Chromium; 25 Mn 54.938 Manganese; 26 Fe 55.845 Iron; 27 Co 58.933 Cobalt; 28 Ni 58.693 Nickel; 29 Cu 63.546 Cooper; 30 Zn 65.39 Zinc

40 Zr 91.224 Zirconium; 41 Nb 92.906 Niobium; 42 Mo 95.94 Molybdenum; 43 Tc 98 Technetium; 44 Ru 101.07 Ruthenium; 45 Rh 102.91 Rhodium; 46 Pd 106.42 Palladium; 47 Ag 107.87 Silver; 48 Cd 112.41 Cadmium

72 Hf 178.49 Hafnium; 73 Ta 180.95 Tantalum; 74 W 183.84 Tungsten; 75 Re 186.21 Rhenium; 76 Os 190.23 Osmium; 77 Ir 192.22 Iridium; 78 Pt 195.08 Platinum; 79 Au 196.97 Gold; 80 Hg 200.59 Mercury

104 Rf 261 Rutherfordium; 105 Db 262 Dubnium; 106 Sg 266 Seaborgium; 107 Bh 264 Bohrium; 108 Hs 269 Hassium; 109 Mt 268 Meitnerium; 110 Uun 271 Ununnilium; 111 Uuu 272 Unununium; 112 Uub 1.0079 Ununbium

5 B 10.811 Boron; 6 C 12.011 Carbon; 7 N 14.007 Nitrogen; 8 O 15.999 Oxygen; 9 F 18.998 Fluorine; 2 He 4.0026 Helium

13 Al 26.982 Aluminium; 14 Si 28.086 Silicon; 15 P 30.974 Phosphorus; 16 S 32.065 Sulfur; 17 Cl 35.453 Chlorine; 10 Ne 20.180 Neon

31 Ga 69.723 Gallium; 32 Ge 1.0079 Germanium; 33 As 74.992 Arsenic; 34 Se 78.96 Selenium; 35 Br 79.904 Bromine; 18 Ar 39.948 Argon

49 In 114.82 Indium; 50 Sn 118.71 Tin; 51 Sb 121.76 Antimony; 52 Te 127.60 Tellurium; 53 I 126.90 Iodine; 36 Kr 83.80 Krypton

81 Tl 204.38 Thallium; 82 Pb 207.2 Lead; 83 Bi 208.98 Bismuth; 84 Po 209 Polonium; 85 At 210 Astatine; 54 Xe 131.29 Xenon

113 Uut Ununtrium; 114 Uuq 289 Ununquadium; 115 Uup Ununpentium; 116 Uuh Ununhexium; 117 Uus Ununseptium; 86 Rn 222 Radon

118 Uuo Ununoctium

Lanthanide series: 57 La 138.91 Lanthanide; 58 Ce 140.12 Cerium; 59 Pr 140.91 Praseodymium; 60 Nd 144.24 Neodymium; 61 Pm 145 Promethium; 62 Sm 150.36 Samarium; 63 Eu 151.96 Europium; 64 Gd 157.25 Gadolinium; 65 Tb 158.93 Terbium; 66 Dy 162.5 Dysprosium; 67 Ho 164.93 Holmium; 68 Er 1.0079 Erbium; 69 Tm 168.93 Thulium; 70 Yb 173.04 Ytterbium; 71 Lu 1.0079 Lutetium

Actinide series: 89 Ac 227 Actinide; 90 Th 232.04 Thorium; 91 Pa 231.04 Protactinium; 92 U 238.03 Uranium; 93 Np 237 Neptunium; 94 Pu 244 Plutonium; 95 Am 243 Americium; 96 Cm 247 Curium; 97 Bk 247 Berkelium; 98 Cf 251 Californium; 99 Es 252 Einsteinium; 100 Fm 257 Fermium; 101 Md 258 Mendelevium; 102 No 259 Nobelium; 103 Lr 1.0079 Lawrencium

AA

Pitting Edema Scale

Pitting edema is a subjective evaluation in which a finger pressing gently into the skin over an accumulation of fluid will result in a temporary depression. Under normal conditions, the depression quickly rebounds when the pressure is released. Four scales (from +1 to +4) are used to differentiate the degree of edema, either by the depth of depression or time needed for rebound. The figure below uses the depth of depression to assign a scale. Some practitioners use the time needed for rebound to assign a scale (e.g., 1–3 seconds for +1; 15 to 20 seconds for +4). As methods are based on subjective evaluations, practitioners should describe objectively the observation and the location of edema.

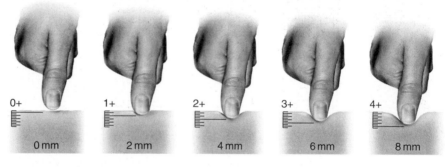

0+ No pitting edema
1+ Mild pitting edema. 2 mm depression that disappears rapidly.
2+ Moderate pitting edema. 4 mm depression that disappears in 10–15 seconds.
3+ Moderately severe pitting edema. 6 mm depression that may last more than 1 minute.
4+ Severe pitting edema. 8 mm depression that can last more than 2 minutes.

REFERENCE

faculty.msmc.edu

BB
Pressure Conversion Table

Atmosphere	cm H$_2$0	mm Hg	psig	kPa
1	1033	760	14.7	101.325
0.000968	1	0.735	0.0142	0.09806
0.001316	1.36	1	0.0193	0.1333
0.068	70.31	51.7	1	6.895
0.00987	10.197	7.501	0.145	1

REFERENCE

http://www.onlineconversion.com/pressure.htm

CC
Ramsay Sedation Scale

The Ramsay Sedation Scale (Ramsay) is a simple assessment to evaluate the degree of sedation. The scale ranges from 1 (patient awake, anxious, agitated, or restless) to 6 (no response to gentle glabellar tap or loud noises).

Sedation scales are generally not suitable for paralyzed patients. Autonomic signs such as tachycardia, diaphoresis, hypertension, and lacrimation should be noted as they may suggest inadequate sedation or pain control.

LEVEL OF RESPONSE (1 TO 6)

1. Awake and anxious, agitated, or restless
2. Awake, cooperative, accepting ventilation, oriented, tranquil
3. Awake; responds only to verbal commands
4. Asleep; brisk response to light, gentle glabellar (between the eyebrows) tap or loud noise
5. Asleep; sluggish response to gentle glabellar tap or loud noise stimulus
6. Asleep; no response to gentle glabellar tap or loud noise stimulus

REFERENCE

Modified from Ramsay, M., Savege, T., Simpson, B.R.J., et al. (1974). "Controlled sedation with alphaxalone/alphadolone." *BMJ, 2*:920, 656–669.

DD
Revised Sedation Scale

The Revised Sedation Scale (RSS) uses three categories to assess the appropriate level of sedation needed for patients in the ICU. These categories are Agitation, Alertness, and Respiration. RSS establishes a sedation goal for patient management and weaning from mechanical ventilation.

One category of RSS assesses the patient's respiration. RSS is therefore suitable for mechanically ventilated patients. A *low* or *decreasing* RSS value correlates with sedation.

Sedation scales are generally not suitable for paralyzed patients. Autonomic signs such as tachycardia, diaphoresis, hypertension, and lacrimation should be noted as they may suggest inadequate sedation or pain control.

RSS PATIENT CLASSIFICATION

1. Acutely ill (weaning not a goal); sedation goal 5–9
2. Chronic ventilated patient (weaning not a goal); sedation goal 6–9
3. Nonventilated patient; sedation goal 7–9
4. Ventilated patient being weaned; sedation goal 7–10

Category	Scale	Description
Agitation	1	Unresponsive to commands/physical stimulation
	2	Appropriate response to physical stimuli/calm
	3	Mild anxiety/delirium/agitation
	4	Moderate anxiety/delirium/agitation
	5	Severe anxiety/delirium/agitation
Alertness	1	Difficult to arouse; eyes remain closed
	2	Mostly sleeping; eyes closed
	3	Dozing intermittently; arouses easily
	4	Awake, calm
	5	Wide awake, hyper-alert
Respiration	1	Intubated, no spontaneous effort
	2	Respirations even, synchronized with ventilator
	3	Mild dyspnea/tachypnea, occasional asynchrony*
	4	Frequent dyspnea/tachypnea, ventilator asynchrony
	5	Sustained, severe dyspnea/tachypnea

*Asynchrony not corrected by ventilator setting adjustments

REFERENCE

Laing. (1992). medscape.com/viewarticle/587336_appendix1

EE

Richmond Agitation and Sedation Scale

The Richmond Agitation and Sedation Scale (RASS) has been tested on ventilated and non-ventilated patients in different ICUs. It provides more detailed agitation and sedation categories than the Ramsay Sedation Scale (Ramsay) and the Sedation Agitation Scale (SAS). RASS assesses the patient's reaction to ET tube and ventilator. It is therefore suitable for mechanically ventilated patients. *Negative* RASS values correlate with degrees of sedation.

Sedation scales are generally not suitable for paralyzed patients. Autonomic signs such as tachycardia, diaphoresis, hypertension, and lacrimation should be noted as they may suggest inadequate sedation or pain control.

RASS PROCEDURE (USE TABLE)

1. Observe patient. If calm, score 0. If restless or agitated, evaluate and score from +1 to +4.
2. If not alert, call patient by name in clear, loud voice and ask patient to look at speaker. Repeat once if necessary. Evaluate and score from −1 to −3.
3. If no response to voice, then physically stimulate patient. Evaluate and score from −4 to −5.

Score	Term	Description
+4	Combative	Overly combative/violent. Danger to staff.
+3	Very agitated	Pulls/removes tubes or catheters. Aggressive.
+2	Agitated	Nonpurposeful movement. Not synchronous with ventilator.
+1	Restless	Anxious, but movement not aggressive/violent.
0	Alert and calm	
−1	Drowsy	Sustained awakening (>10 sec) with eye contact to voice.
−2	Light sedation	Briefly awakens (<10 sec) with eye contact to voice.
−3	Moderate sedation	Movement to voice, but no eye contact.
−4	Deep sedation	No response to voice. Movement to physical stimulation.
−5	Unarousable	No response to voice or physical stimulation.

REFERENCE

Sessler; medscape.com/viewarticle/587336_appendix1

FF

Sedation Agitation Scale

The sedation agitation scale (SAS) provides more detailed agitation categories than the Ramsay Sedation Scale (Ramsay). The SAS assesses pulling or biting at the ET tube. It is therefore suitable for mechanically ventilated patients. A *low* or *decreasing* SAS value correlates with sedation.

Sedation scales are generally not suitable for paralyzed patients. Autonomic signs such as tachycardia, diaphoresis, hypertension, and lacrimation should be noted as they may suggest inadequate sedation or pain control.

LEVEL OF RESPONSE (7 TO 1)

7. Dangerous agitation (e.g., pulling at ET tube, trying to remove catheters, climbing over bed rail, striking at staff)
6. Very agitated (e.g., biting at ET tube, requiring physical restraints)
5. Agitated (anxious or mildly agitated, trying to sit up, calms down to verbal instructions)
4. Calm and cooperative (calm, awakens easily, follows commands)
3. Sedated (difficult to arouse, awakens to verbal stimuli or gentle shaking but drifts off again, follows simple commands)
2. Very sedated (arouses to physical stimuli but does not communicate or follow commands may move spontaneously)
1. Unarousable (minimal or no response to noxious stimuli, does not communicate or follow commands)

REFERENCE

Riker; medscape.com/viewarticle/587336_appendix1

GG
Therapeutic Blood Levels of Selected Drugs

Drug	Therapeutic Level	Toxic Level
Alcohols		
Ethanol	0.1 g/dL	100 mg/dL
Methanol	—	20 mg/dL
Antibiotics		
Amikacin	20–25 mcg/mL	35 mcg/mL
SI Units	34–43 µmol/L	60 µmol/L
Gentamicin	4–8 mcg/mL	12 mcg/mL
SI units	8.4–16.8 µmol/L	25.1 µmol/L
Kanamycin	20–25 mcg/mL	35 mcg/mL
SI units	42–52 µmol/L	73 µmol/L
Streptomycin	25–30 mcg/mL	>30 mcg/mL
SI Units	—	—
Tobramycin	2–8 mcg/mL	12 mcg/mL
SI units	4–17 µmol/L	25 µmol/L
Anticonvulsants		
Barbiturates		
Amobarbital	7 mcg/mL	30 mcg/mL
SI units	30 µmol/L	132 µmol/L
Pentobarbital	4 mcg/ml	15 mcg/ml
SI units	18 µmol/L	66 µmol/L
Phenobarbital	10 mcg/mL	>55 mcg/mL
SI units	43 µmol/L	>230 µmol/L
Primidone	1 mcg/ml	>10 µmol/L
SI units	4 µmol/L	>45 µmol/L
Benzodiazepines		
Clonazepam	5–70 ng/mL	>70 ng/mL
SI units	55–222 µmol/L	>222 µmol/L
Diazepam (Valium)	5–70 ng/mL	>70 ng/mL
SI units	0.01–0.25 µmol/L	>0.25 µmol/L
Hydantoins		
Phenytoin (Dilantin)	10–18 mcg/mL	>20 mcg/mL
SI units	40–80 µmol/L	>80 µmol/L

Drug	Therapeutic Level	Toxic Level
Succinimides		
Euthosuximide (Zarontin)	40–80 mcg/mL	100 mcg/mL
SI units	283–566 µmol/L	708 µmol/L
Other		
Carbamazepine (Tegretol)	2–10 mcg/mL	12 mcg/mL
SI units	8–42 µmol/L	50 µmol/L
Valproic acid (Depakene)	50–100 mcg/mL	>100 mcg/mL
SI units	350–700 µmol/L	>700 µmol/L
Bronchodilators		
Aminophylline/theophylline	10–18 mcg/mL	20 mcg/ml,
Cardiac Drugs		
Disopyramide (Norpace)	2–4.5 mcg/mL	>9 mcg/mL
SI units	5.9 µmol/L	26 µmol/L
Quinidine	2.4–5 mcg/mL	>6 mcg/mL
SI units	7–15 µmol/L	>18 µmol/L
Procainamide (Pronestyl)	7–15 mcg/mL	>12 mcg/mL
SI units	17–35 µmol/L	>50 µmol/L
Lidocaine	2–6 mcg/mL	>9 mcg/mL
SI units	8–25 µmol/L	>38 µmol/L
Bretylium	5–10 mg/kg	30 mg/kg
Verapamil	5–10 mg/kg	>15 mg/kg
Diltiazem	50–200 ng/mL	>200 ng/mL
Nifedipine	5–10 mg/kg	90 mg/kg
Digitoxin	10–25 ng/mL	30 ng/mL
SI units	13–33 nmol/L	39 nmol/L
Digoxin	0.5–2 ng/mL	>2.5 ng/mL
SI units	0.6–2.5 nmol/L	>3.0 nmol/L
Phenytoin (Dilantin)	10–18 mcg/mL	>20 mcg/mL
SI units	40–71 µmol/L	>80 µmol/L
Quinidine	2.3–5 mcg/mL	>5 mcg/mL
SI units	7–15 µmol/L	>15 µmol/L
Narcotics		
Codeine		>0.005 mg/dL
SI units		>17 nmol/dL
Hydromorphone (Dilaudid)		>0.1 mg/dL
SI units		>350 nmol/L
Methadone		>0.2 mg/dL
SI units		6.46 µmol/L
Meperidine (Demerol)		0.5 mg/dL
SI units		20 µmol/L
Morphine		0.005 mg/dL
Psychiatrics		
Amitriptyline (Elavil)	100–250 ng/mL	>300 ng/mL
SI units	361–902 nmol/L	>1083 nmol/L
Imiprimine (Tofranil)	100–250 ng/mL	>300 ng/mL
SI units	357–898 nmol/L	>1071 nmol/L
Lithium (Lithonate)	0.8–1.4 mEq/L	1.5 mEq/L
SI units	0.8–1.4 µmol/L	1.5 µmol/L

Drug	Therapeutic Level	Toxic Level
Salicylates		
Aspirin	2–20 mg/dL	>30 mg/dL
SI units	0.1–1.4 mmol/L	>2.1 mmol/L
Other		
Acetaminophen	0–25 mcg/mL	>150 mcg/ml
SI units	0–170 µmol/L	>1000 µmol/L
Bromides	75–150 mg/dL	>150 mg/dL
SI units	7–15 mmol/L	>15 mmol/L
Prochlorperazine	0.5 mcg/mL	1.0 mcg/mL

HH
Weaning Criteria

Category	Examples	Values
Ventilatory Criteria	Spontaneous breathing trial	Tolerates 30 to 120 min.
	$PaCO_2$	<50 mm Hg with normal pH
	Vital capacity	>10 to 15 mL/Kg
	Spontaneous V_T	>5 to 8 mL/Kg
	Spontaneous f	<30/min
	f/V_T (rapid shallow breathing index)	<100 breaths/min/L
	Minute ventilation	<10 L with normal ABG
Oxygenation Criteria	PaO_2 without *PEEP*	>60 mm Hg at F_IO_2 up to 0.4
	PaO_2 with *PEEP*	>100 mm Hg at F_IO_2 up to 0.4
	SaO_2	>90% at F_IO_2 up to 0.4
	Q_s/Q_T	<20%
	$P_{(A-a)}O_2$	<350 mm Hg at F_IO_2 of 1.0
	PaO_2/F_IO_2	>200 mm Hg
Pulmonary Reserve	Maximal voluntary ventilation	2x min vent at F_IO_2 up to 0.4
	Maximal inspiratory pressure	>−20 to −30 cm H_2O in 20 sec.
Pulmonary Measurements	Static compliance	>30 mL/cm H_2O
	Airway resistance	Improving trend
	V_D/V_T	<60% (while intubated)

Bibliography

"Apgar Scoring," Coastal Valley EMS Agency, last modified July 2006, http://www
.sonoma-county.org/cvrems/resources/pdf/guidelines/9405.pdf.

"Apgar Scoring for Newborns," Childbirth.org, accessed August 4, 2011, http://www
.childbirth.org/articles/apgar.html.

Banner, M., Downs, B., Kirby, R., Smith, R., Boysen, P., & Lampotang, M., "Effects
on Expiratory Flow Resistance on Inspiratory Work of Breathing," *Chest Journal*
93/4 (1988): 795–799, accessed August 4, 2011, http://chestjournal.chestpubs.org/
content/93/4/795.full.pdf.

Barnes, T. A., et al. (1993). *Core Textbook of Respiratory Care Practice.* St. Louis, MO:
Mosby-Year Book.

Bjornson, C. L., et al. (1992). *N Engl J Med, 351,* 1306–1313.

"Blood Pressure, Neonatal Handbook" The Royal Children's Hospital, accessed
August 4, 2011, http://www.rch.org.au/nets/handbook/index/cfm?doc_id=450.

"BMI Calculator-Harris Benedict Equation," accessed August 24, 2001, http://www
.bmi-calculator.net/bmr-calculator/harris-benedict-equation/.

"BMR Calculator," Calculators Live, accessed August 4, 2011, http://www
.calculatorslive.com/BMR-Calculator.aspx.

Burton, G. G., et al. (1997). *Respiratory Care: A Guide to Clinical Practice.* 4th ed.
Philadelphia, PA: Lippincott Williams & Wilkins.

Bustin, D. (1986). *Hemodynamic Monitoring for Critical Care.* Norwalk, CT:
Appleton-Century-Crofts.

Chang, D. W. (2006). *Clinical Application of Mechanical Ventilation.* 3rd ed. Clifton
Park, NY: Delmar Cengage Learning.

Chatburn, R. L., et al. (2009). *Handbook for Health Care Research.* 2nd ed. Sudbury,
MA: Jones & Bartlett Publishers.

Colbert, B. J. et al. (2011). *Integrated Cardiopulmonary Pharmacology.* 3rd ed. Upper
Saddle River, New Jersey: Pearson.

"Croup: What You Need to Know," About.com Pediatrics, last modified June 16,
2011, http://www.pediatrics.about.com/cs/commoninfections/a/croup.htm.

Des Jardins, T. R. *Cardiopulmonary Anatomy and Physiology: Essentials
for Respiratory Care.* 5th ed. Clifton Park, NY: Delmar Cengage Learning, 2007.

"Dosage Calculations," DosageHelp, accessed August 4, 2011, http://www.Dosagehelp
.com.

Dubois, E. F. (1924). *Basal Metabolism in Health and Disease.* Philadelphia: Lea and
Febiger.

Dupuis, Y. G. (1992). *Ventilator: Theory and Clinical Application.* 2nd ed. St. Louis,
MO: Mosby-Year Book.

"Endotracheal Tube," Family Practice Notebook, last modified February 20, 2011,
fpnotebook.com/lung/Procedure/EndtrchlTb.htm.

"Faculty Web Site Directory," Mount Saint Mary College, accessed January 2011, faculty.msmc.edu.

"Fagerstrom Test for Nicotine Dependences on Cigarettes," Nova Southeastern University, accessed August 4, 2011, http://nova.edu/gsc/nicotine_risk.html.

Gardenhire, D. S. (2007). *Rau's Respiratory Care Pharmacology*. 7th ed. St. Louis, MO: Mosby-Year Book.

Geelhoed, G. C. (2004). *Pediatr Pulmonol, 20:6*, 362–368.

Gross, L. J. (1985). "Setting cutoff scores on credentialing examinations: a refinement in the Nedelsky Procedure." *Evaluation and the Health Professions 8*: *4*, 469–493.

Hegstad, L. N., et al. (2000). *Essential Drug Dosage Calculations*. 4th ed. Upper Saddle River, NJ: Prentice Hall.

Kacmarek, R. M., et al. (2005). *Essentials of Respiratory Care*. 4th ed. St. Louis, MO: Mosby-Year Book.

Klassen, T. P. (1998). *JAMA, 279:20*, 1629–1632.

Koff, P. B., et al. (2005). *Neonatal and Pediatric Respiratory Care*. 2nd ed. St. Louis, MO: Mosby-Year Book.

Krider, T. M., et al. (1986). *Master Guide for Passing the Respiratory Care Credentialing Exams*. Upper Saddle River, NJ: Prentice Hall, 1998.

Laing, A. S. (1992). "The Applicability of a New Sedation Scale for Intensive Care." *Int Crit Care Nurs 8*(3):149–52.

Madama, V. C. (1998). *Pulmonary Function Testing and Cardiopulmonary Stress Testing*. 2nd ed. Albany, NY: Delmar Publishers.

Malley, W. J. (1990). *Clinical Blood Gases: Application and Noninvasive Alternatives*. Philadelphia, PA: W.B. Saunders.

Nedelsky, L. (1954). "Absolute grading standards for objective tests." *Educational and Psychologic Measurement 14*: 3–19.

Noack, G. (1993). Ventilatory Treatment of Neonates and Infants. Solna, Sweden: Siemens-Elema AB Life Support Systems Division, Marketing Communications.

Pierson, D. J., et al. (1992). *Foundations of Respiratory Care*. New York: Churchill Livingston.

Ramsay, M., Savege, T., Simpson, B. R. J., et al. (1974). "Controlled sedation with alphaxalone/alphadolone." *BMF, 2:920*, 656–669.

"Richmond Agitation-Sedation Scale," Medscape, accessed August 4, 2011, http://www.medscape.com/viewarticle/587336_appendix1.

"Riker Sedation-Agitation Scale," Medscape, accessed August 4, 2011, http://www.medscape.com/viewarticle/587336_appendix1.

Rittichier, K. K. (2000). *Pediatrics, 106(6)*, 1344–1348.

Ruppel, G. L. (2008). *Manual of Pulmonary Function Testing*. 9th ed. St. Louis, MO: Mosby-Year Book.

Shapiro, B. A. et al. (1994). *Clinical Application of Blood Gases*. 5th ed. St. Louis, MO: Mosby-Year Book.

Sorbini, L. A., et al. (1968). "Arterial oxygen tension in relation to age in healthy subjects." *Respiration 25*: 3–13.

Teasdale, G., & Jennett, B. (1974). "Assessment of coma and impaired consciousness: A practical scale," *The Lancet, 304*, 81–84.

Tobin, M. J., et al. (1986). "The pattern of breathing during successful and unsuccessful trials of weaning from mechanical ventilation." *Am Rev Respir Dis 134*: 1111–1118.

Tuckman, R. W. (1993). *Conducting Educational Research.* 4th ed. Boston, MA: Houghton Mifflin Harcourt.

Waisman, Y. (1992). *Pediatrics, 89*:2, 302–306.

Whitaker, K. B., et al. (2001). *Comprehensive Perinatal and Pediatric Respiratory Care.* 3rd ed. Clifton Park, NY: Delmar Cengage Learning.

White, G. C. (2004). *Equipment Theory for Respiratory Care.* 4th ed. Clifton Park, NY: Delmar Cengage Learning.

Wilkins, R. L., et al. (1) (2009). *Clinical Assessment in Respiratory Care.* 6th ed. St. Louis, MO: Mosby-Year Book.

Wilkins, R. L., et al. (2) (2008). *Egan's Fundamental of Respiratory Care.* 9th ed. St. Louis, MO: Mosby-Year Book.

Wojciechwoski, W. V. (1996). *Respiratory Care Sciences: An Integrated Approach.* 2nd ed. Albany, NY: Delmar Cengage Learning.

Wojciechowski, W. V. (2006). *Respiratory Care Sciences: An integrated Approach.* 4th ed. Clifton Park, NY: Delmar Cengage Learning.

Yang, K. L., et al. (1991). "A prospective study of indexes predicting the outcome of trials of weaning from mechanical ventilation." *N Engl J Med 324*: 1445–1450.

Index by Alphabetical Listing